The Integrated Mind

The Integrated Mind

Michael S. Gazzaniga
and Joseph E. LeDoux

Department of Neurology
The New York Hospital
Cornell University Medical College

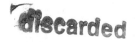
Plenum Press · New York and London

Library of Congress Cataloging in Publication Data

Gazzaniga, Michael S
  The integrated mind.

  Includes bibliographical references and index.
  1. Intellect. 2. Split brain. I. LeDoux, Joseph, joint author. II. Title. [DNLM:
1. Corpus callosum. 2. Neurophysiology. WL307 G291i]
QP398.G39   612'.82   77-20101
ISBN 0-306-31085-6

First Printing—March 1978
Second Printing—April 1979

© 1978 Plenum Press, New York
A Division of Plenum Publishing Corporation
227 West 17th Street, New York, N.Y. 10011

Printed in the United States of America

To DIANA

Preface

In this book we are trying to illuminate the persistent and nagging questions of how mind, life, and the essence of being relate to brain mechanisms. We do that not because we have a commitment to bear witness to the boring issue of reductionism but because we want to know more about what it's all about. How, indeed, does the brain work? How does it allow us to love, hate, see, cry, suffer, and ultimately understand Kepler's laws?

We try to uncover clues to these staggering questions by considering the results of our studies on the bisected brain. Several years back, one of us wrote a book with that title, and the approach was to describe how brain and behavior are affected when one takes the brain apart. In the present book, we are ready to put it back together, and go beyond, for we feel that split-brain studies are now at the point of contributing to an understanding of the workings of the integrated mind.

We are grateful to Dr. Donald Wilson of the Dartmouth Medical School for allowing us to test his patients. We would also like to thank our past and present colleagues, including Richard Nakamura, Gail Risse, Pamela Greenwood, Andy Francis, Andrea Elberger, Nick Brecha, Lynn Bengston, and Sally Springer, who have been involved in various facets of the experimental studies on the bisected brain described in this book. Thanks also to Ellen Friedman, who suffered through the typing and retyping. Finally, and most importantly, our profound thanks to the patients who continue to give their time and energy to our enterprise. They have taught us a lot more about life than we have been able to set forth in this book.

Michael S. Gazzaniga and Joseph E. LeDoux

New York, N.Y.

Contents

1 ▪ The Split Brain and the Integrated Mind   1

Splitting the Brain 1
Splitting the Mind................................... 3
The Split Brain in Transition 6
Opportunities for Validation and Theoretical Advances: The
        Wilson Series 6
References 7

2 ▪ The Nature of Interhemispheric Communication   9

What Transfers and Why? 9
    The Commissural Sensory Window: Its Scope and Limits   11
    What Else Transfers? 13
    The Role of Duplication 17
Where? Clues to Basic Principles 19
Visual Transfer: Variability, Specificity, and Plasticity in
        Brain Organization 19
    The Human Anterior Commissure: Individual Differences
        in Visual Transfer 20
    Comparative Variability in the Transfer Mechanism 23
    Neural Specificity 27
Laterality Effects in Somesthesis: Clues to Somatosensory
        Organization, Cuing Strategies, and
        Shifting Circuits 29
    Somatosensory Organization 30
    Human Studies 31
    Animal Studies 36
Conclusion 39
References 39

*3 ▪ Cerebral Lateralization and Hemisphere
        Specialization: Facts and Theory*   45

Cerebral Lateralization: The Facts   46
Hemisphere Specialization   47
Manipulospatial Aspects of Cerebral Lateralization   49
    The Nature of Manipulospatial Activities   55
    The Neural Substrate of Manipulospatiality   56
    The Language–Manipulospatial Relationship   59
    Competition for Synaptic Space   60
    Origins   62
Perceptual Processing and Cerebral Lateralization   63
    Split-Brain Studies   64
    Normal Studies   67
    Clinical Studies of Visual Recognition   68
Loose Ends   69
Conclusions   71
References   72

4 ▪ Brain and Language   77

Language Development and Lateralization   78
Right-Hemisphere Language in the Left-Dominant
        Population?   83
Language and Praxis   91
Artificial and Natural Language   92
Psycholinguistics and the Brain Sciences   96
Language and Memory   97
References   98

5 ▪ Brain and Intelligence   103

Cortical Equipotentiality and Interhemispheric Dynamics . . .   103
Mass Action   104
    How Smart Is the Half-Brain?   105
    Cognitive Cost of Commissurotomy   109
    The Neurology of Intelligence   115
References   117

6 ▪ *Brain, Imagery, and Memory*   121

How Visual Is Visual Imagery? 121
Memory 124
    Basic Issues in Learning and Memory: Errors, Rewards,
        and Motives 125
    Multiple Neural Coding 130
    Multidimensionality of Experience and Information Storage 132
    Implications for a Theory of Memory 135
References 138

7 ▪ *On the Mechanisms of Mind*   141

Split Consciousness 142
Verbal Attribution and the Sociology of Mind 146
Emotion and Consciousness 151
Why the Need for Consonance? 155
    Cross-Cuing 157
    Developmental Aspects 158
The Multiple Self and Free Will 159
References 161

Author Index 163

Subject Index 167

The Split Brain and the Integrated Mind

The foremost objective of the brain sciences is, of course, to determine the relation between mind and brain. Our particular approach to the problem focuses on the neurological and psychological consequences of disrupting the dynamics of interhemispheric interactions, and in this first chapter we will briefly consider the historical antecedents of our current studies of the split brain.

SPLITTING THE BRAIN

The corpus callosum, the largest fiber tract in the human brain, contains over 200 million neurons that interconnect the left and right cerebral hemispheres (Figure 1). As late as the 1940s, the callosum was considered an enigma by neurologists and neurosurgeons and was the structure discussed most often when an example was sought to show how little was known about the brain. The general consensus was that the "great cerebral commissure" could be sectioned and destroyed without apparent consequence.

It was in this context that the original experiments on the split brain were carried out in the cat by Ronald Myers and Roger Sperry at the University of Chicago. Myers had successfully developed the surgical technique of splitting the optic chiasm, thereby

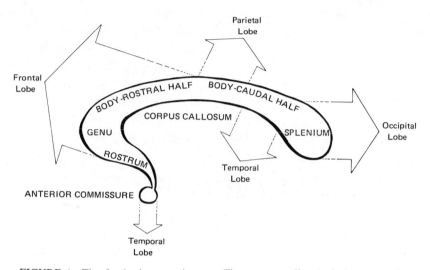

FIGURE 1. The forebrain commissures. The corpus callosum is known to be functionally divided in a manner that finds the interhemispheric fibers coursing through the posterior area, or splenium, to be projected primarily to the occipital lobe. As shown, the body of the callosum projects to the parietal lobe, and the anterior regions interconnect the frontal lobes. The temporal lobe is interconnected via the anterior commissure and the caudal parts of the body of the callosum.

allowing visual information presented to the right eye to be exclusively projected to the right hemisphere and input to the left eye to be similarly directed to the left hemisphere. He then observed that when such cats were monocularly trained on visual discrimination problems, the animals could perform the task using the untrained eye alone. In other words, surgical section of the optic chiasm failed to prevent interocular transfer, and this could only mean that the interocular integration had taken place somewhere inside the brain. The most obvious neurological candidate for the next surgery was the corpus callosum. The surgical and behavioral procedures were carried out, and this study, which gave birth to the split-brain paradigm, demonstrated that following midline division of the optic chiasm and corpus callosum of the cat, discriminations trained to one half of the brain left the other side naive.

Still, however, these results stood in marked contrast to the earlier studies of A. J. Akelaitis, who had examined a series of some 26 patients with the corpus callosum and anterior commissure completely or partially sectioned in an effort to control the interhemispheric spread of epileptic seizures. In an extensive series of studies, he purported to show that sectioning these structures did not result in any significant neurological or psychological sequels. This point was made—and it emerged as the dominant view—even though there were several contradictory reports in the literature showing disconnection effects as a result of having the callosum sectioned or rendered nonfunctional by a tumor or the like. It was also generally considered that cutting the callosum did not, in fact, help control epilepsy.

Then, in 1960, Dr. Joseph Bogen, who at the time was a resident at White Memorial Hospital in Los Angeles, proposed, after a careful review of Akelaitis's studies, that the brain could be split for the purpose of controlling the interhemispheric spread of epilepsy. His hunch that the surgery should work proved largely correct. It was his first patient, W.J., that was extensively studied both pre- and postoperatively on a host of psychological tests that were devised at the California Institute of Technology. In subsequent studies of W. J. and other patients in the Bogen series, a variety of striking and dramatic effects were observed [1].

SPLITTING THE MIND

One of the immediate and compelling consequences of brain bisection was that the interhemispheric exchange of information was totally disrupted, so that visual, tactual, proprioceptive, auditory, and olfactory information presented to one hemisphere could be processed and dealt with in that half-brain, but these activities would go on outside the realm of awareness of the other half-cerebrum. Thus, the data confirmed the earlier animal work by Myers and Sperry but were, in a sense, more dramatic, in that only processes ongoing in the left hemisphere could be verbally described by the patients, since it is the left hemisphere that normally possesses the natural language and speech mechanisms. Thus, for example, if a word (such as *spoon*) was flashed in the left visual field, which is exclusively projected to the right hemisphere in man (Figure 2), the subject, when asked, would say, "I did not see anything," but then subsequently would be able, with the left hand, to retrieve the correct object from a series of objects

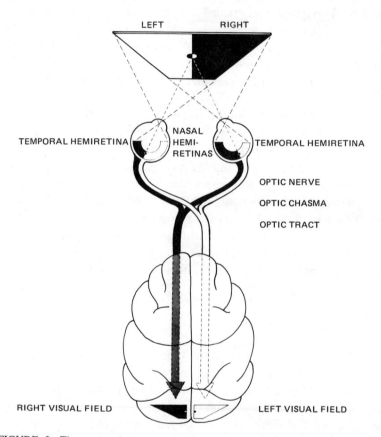

FIGURE 2. The anatomical relationship that must be clearly understood in a consideration of visual studies on the bisected brain are shown here. Because of the distribution of fibers in the optic system, information presented to each eye is projected almost equally to both hemispheres. In order to assure that information is presented to only one hemisphere, the subject must fixate a point. As a consequence of the anatomical arrangement shown here, information projected to the right visual field goes only to the left hemisphere, and vice-versa.

placed out of view (Figure 3). Furthermore, if the experimenter asked, "What do you have in your hand?" the subject would typically say, "I don't know." Here again, the talking hemisphere did not know. It did not see the picture, nor did it have access to the stereognostic (touch) information from the left hand, which is also exclusively projected to the right hemisphere. Yet, clearly, the right half-brain knew the answer, because it reacted appropriately to the correct stimulus.

That each half-brain could process information outside the realm of awareness of the other raised the intriguing possibility that the mechanisms of consciousness were doubly represented following brain bisection. The implications of this controversial possibility were far-reaching and attracted the interest of philosophers and scientists alike. However, while the conscious properties of the talking hemisphere were apparent, the view that the mute hemisphere was also deserving of conscious status was widely criticized and generally rejected. Consequently, subsequent studies focused on elucidating the nature of information processing in the right hemisphere.

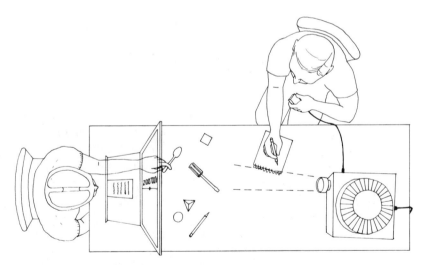

FIGURE 3. The basic testing arrangement used for the examination of lateralized visual and stereognostic functions. See text for explanation.

THE SPLIT BRAIN IN TRANSITION

A variety of studies moved ahead to show that the right hemisphere possessed superior skills on some nonverbal tasks, such as in drawing and copying designs and in arranging items to construct complex patterns. In a general way, the left half-brain seemed to be the hemisphere of choice for verbal processing, with the right hemisphere excelling in certain nonverbal situations.

Then, in the late 1960s and early 1970s, the basic claims concerning hemisphere functioning underwent a radical change. There arose a barrage of popular and overdramatized accounts of the uniqueness of mind left and mind right. These representations of the implications of the split-brain observations gave rise to a cult-like following and were largely written by people who had never seen a patient, but they were fed, in part, by new studies carried out by those directly involved in the experimental enterprise. We believe that these "pop" versions of hemisphere function are in error, and a good deal of the business of this book is to reestablish a basic, sober framework for considering studies on cerebral commissurotomy.

OPPORTUNITIES FOR VALIDATION AND THEORETICAL ADVANCES: THE WILSON SERIES

In early 1970, Donald Wilson of the Dartmouth Medical School commenced a new series of commissure-sectioned patients[2]. Using a different surgical approach, Wilson, in the first phase of the series, variably sectioned the entire corpus callosum and anterior commissure. In the second and current phase, only the corpus callosum is sectioned, with the anterior commissure explicitly left intact[3].

The neuropsychological assessment of these patients, both pre- and postoperatively, is a unique research opportunity that has fallen to our laboratory (Figure 4). The results of the studies thus far completed, as well as the results of a variety of independent studies, are presented in the following pages. These data allow for

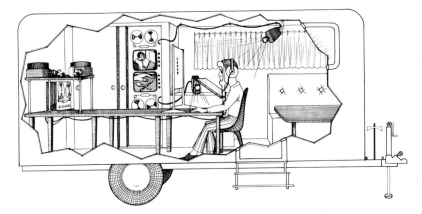

FIGURE 4. Testing of the Wilson series of patients has involved logistical as well as scientific considerations. Most of the patients live in the greater New England area, and each is privately tested in our specially designed mobile unit. Tachistoscopic, dichotic, and assorted other testing procedures are carried out and recorded on video tape. Figure reprinted from M. S. Gazzaniga, G. L. Risse, S. P. Springer, E. Clark, and D. H. Wilson, 1975, Psychologic and neurologic consequences of partial and complete cerebral commissurotomy, *Neurology 25:*10–15.

what we feel are new interpretations of inter- and intrahemispheric mechanisms, but more importantly, these data allow us to extend the implications of split-brain studies beyond lateralization and toward an understanding of the nature and mechanisms of the integrated mind.

REFERENCES

1. M. S. Gazzaniga, 1970, *The Bisected Brain,* New York, Appleton-Century-Crofts.
2. D. H. Wilson, A. G. Reeves, M. S. Gazzaniga, and C. Culver, 1977, Cerebral commissurotomy for the control of intractable seizures, *Neurology* 27:708–715.
3. D. H. Wilson, A. Reeves, and M. S. Gazzaniga, Corpus callosotomy for the control of intractable epilepsy, *J. Neurosurg.,* submitted.

The Nature of Interhemispheric Communication

The human brain is organized so that two potentially independent mental systems exist side by side. When separated by the slice of a surgeon's knife, each resulting half-brain possesses its own capacities for learning, emoting, thinking, and acting. Yet, with the forebrain commissures intact, these potentially independent neural spheres work together to maintain mental unity.

In this chapter, we explore the fascinating role of the corpus callosum and the anterior commissure in the maintenance of mental unity. Our goal is to specify the essence of commissural function by elucidating the "what," "why," and "where" of interhemispheric communication. We begin this quest billions of years ago in the sea.

WHAT TRANSFERS AND WHY?

A paleoniscid swims in its prehistoric aquarium in search of food. A suitable prey is detected in the right visual field, moving rapidly to the left. Before the primitive vertebrate can change its course, the prey crosses the visual midline and enters the left visual field. Because the optic projections of the fish are crossed, the right visual field is seen by the right eye and the left half-brain, and vice versa. Does this mean that when the prey moves out of one visual field and into the other, the neural control over the chase switches from an informed to a naive half-brain? Hardly!

The commissural system (which is more accurately called a system of decussations in nonmammals) provides each half-brain with a copy of the sensory world directly observed by the other hemisphere. It is by way of this incredible feat of neural engineering that the integrated organism responds to sensory stimulation selectively channeled to one half of the brain. This ancient vertebrate blueprint is as relevant for the fish as it is for man.

Consider case D.H. Prior to surgery, D.H. could, without the aid of vision, find an object with one hand that had only been felt by the other. After surgery, however, he could no longer accomplish this simple task. Tactual information in the left hand and the right hemisphere remained isolated from the right hand and the left hemisphere. Yet, when a visual stimulus, such as the picture of an apple, was lateralized to either hemisphere, either hand could manually retrieve the apple, unaided by visual exploration. This unique phenomenon is attributable to the fact that D.H.'s anterior commissure was intentionally spared by the surgeon. Because this interhemispheric bundle contains visual fibers but not somatosensory fibers, D.H. was tactually split but not visually split. So, regardless of which hemisphere saw the apple directly, both ulti-

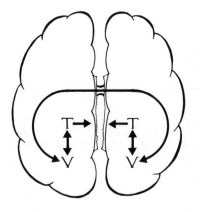

FIGURE 5. The specificity of functions in the fully developed cerebral commissures is quite remarkable. Surgical section of the corpus callosum in case D.H. found visual information transferring through the remaining anterior commissure. Tactile information does not transfer. Predictably, however, visual-tactile matches can be carried out (see text).

mately had access to the visual input. As a consequence, either hemisphere could tactually retrieve the apple in response to the lateralized visual cue.

These observations suggest that the commissures shuttle sensory messages between the hemispheres, and this conclusion is consistent with the physiological properties of the interhemispheric pathways[1-8]. Tactual information from the left hand reaches the right hemisphere by direct sensory channels but reaches the left hemisphere by commissural channels. Similarly, the contralateral visual field is represented in a hemisphere directly, while the ipsilateral representation is by way of the commissures. This phenomenon leads us to ask whether the sensory sphere created by commissural transmission is as complete as the sphere set up more directly. Alternatively, is information lost during interhemispheric transfer?

The Commissural Sensory Window: Its Scope and Limits

Several lines of evidence have suggested that the information reaching a hemisphere by way of the commissural sensory window is limited relative to direct sensory channels. The first claim came from Myers, who found that the monocular training of optic-chiasm–sectioned cats, followed by section of the corpus callosum, leaves the untrained hemisphere capable of performing "simple" but not more "complex" tasks[9-12]. The inference from these studies has been that the commissures serve as a filter that transmits limited information. While simple visual cues leak across during training, more complex information remains lateralized.

Comparable experiments on primates have demonstrated that, except under special conditions[13], the unilateral training of one hemisphere results in the formation of engrams in both hemispheres, regardless of the discriminative complexity of the stimuli[14, 15]. These studies have suggested, however, that the commissurally established memory lacks the strength of the engram formed in the trained hemisphere. While on the surface such results point to commissural transmission limits, control tests have suggested that the deficits seen are performance rather than transfer deficits[14], a finding that highlights the methodological inadequacy of using a learning measure as an index of sensory transfer.

When transfer is studied in human subjects, where no training as such is needed to measure interhemispheric communication, complete transfer is found. Again, consider D.H., our partial-commissurotomy case who is tactually split but is visually intact. When complex visual stimuli are presented exclusively to the left visual field, D.H. is capable of giving a running verbalization[16]. Here, he uses the speech mechanisms of his left hemisphere to describe visual images seen directly by the right hemisphere alone.

Clearly, then, it would seem that Myers's experiments on the cat and the inferences from them about the nature of the commissural code are inappropriate for monkey and man, and methodological considerations render the conclusions, even for the cat, somewhat dubious[17]. The behavioral data thus fail to clearly demonstrate commissural transmission limits and in fact suggest that the evidence for such limits is more apparent than real.

On the other hand, it is commonly argued that there is a physiological basis for the idea that there are severe limits on the commissural transfer mechanism. The argument is that while the contralateral visual field is fully represented in each hemisphere, the representation of the ipsilateral field, which is provided by the splenium of the callosum, is equivalent to a narrow slit near the visual midline[5-14]. This argument is based on the finding that the bilateral cells in the visual cortex that give rise to and receive callosal fibers have very narrow ipsilateral receptive fields, subtending only a few degrees of visual arc[1-5]. However, retinal acuity drops rapidly within a few degrees of arc from the fovea, and this decrease corresponds with the decrease in density of cones with increasing lateral distance from the fovea[18]. Thus, although the callosal representation of the ipsilateral hemifield is limited relative to the size of the whole hemifield, it is more than sufficient to accommodate that portion of the visual field seen with the greatest acuity. Furthermore, visual commissural connections also arise and terminate in the inferior temporal cortex, where bilateral cells have been found that extend more than 35° into the ipsilateral visual field[19]. Thus, it is apparent that commissural fibers are capable of transmitting as much information as can be accurately perceived in the periphery (if not more). In addition, eye movements are continuously directing relevant aspects of the visual world to the cone-dense and commissurally rich foveal region.

These observations leave us, on the whole, doubting whether there are severe limits in the capacity of the commissures to transmit sensory information from one half-brain to the other. In fact, the data actually suggest that the view of the world created in a hemisphere by direct sensory channels is largely duplicated in the contralateral hemisphere by way of the commissural sensory window. With this conclusion, we leave the topic of sensory transfer and turn to the question of what else transfers.

What Else Transfers?

The idea that engrams themselves might transfer dates back to the pioneering studies of Myers and Sperry[20]. When these investigators first identified the forebrain commissures as the neural system subserving interhemispheric communication, they described the effect as the ''interhemispheric transfer of training,'' which implies that it is the fruit of training—the engram for the task—that transfers. Yet, it should be obvious that the simpler concept of sensory transfer readily accounts for the data. When one hemisphere is trained and the commissures are intact, the trained hemisphere learns by direct sensory exposure, while the untrained hemisphere learns by commissural sensory exposure. Thus, the transfer-of-training notion reflects the methodological conditions under which the phenomenon was first demonstrated more than it does the underlying neuropsychological reality of interhemispheric communication. Nevertheless, the notion of engram transfer persisted, and the cortical spreading-depression technique emerged in the split-brain setting with the hope that it would demonstrate mobile memories.

Although investigators claim to have demonstrated engram transfer[21], numerous technical and methodological problems haunt the spreading-depression technique[22,23]. In a convincing review,

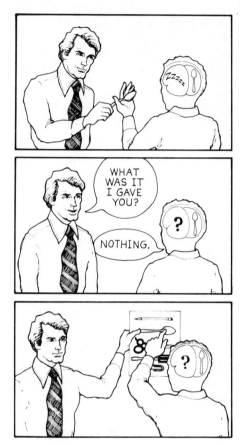

FIGURE 6. During the course of the angiography procedure, sodium amytal is injected. The effect is to anesthetize one half-brain exclusively, but only for a short period of time (see text).

Petrinovich[24] concluded that the contradictory and inconclusive nature of existing studies questions the usefulness of the procedure in precisely elucidating the mechanisms involved in the formation and transfer of memory traces. We could not agree with him more.

Gail Risse has recently approached the problem of engram transfer by running a variation of the traditional carotid amytal tests[25]. These tests are carried out only when cerebral angiography is medically prescribed. In short, the left hemisphere is put to sleep while a specific engram is laid down in the right hemisphere by having the subject tactually palpate a common object with his left hand. When both hemispheres are again awake, the patient is asked to name the object that was in his left hand. The typical response is that he does not know. The patient (or at least his left hemisphere's verbal system) continues to reject all knowledge of the object, even when pressed by the examiner. However, he readily selects the object when provided with a nonverbal means of responding. These data suggest that engrams selectively laid down in one hemisphere remain inaccessible to the awareness of the other half-brain. Only when the "trained" hemisphere is given a chance to respond is there any indication that the information was stored at all. One interpretation of these data is that engrams laid down in one half-brain cannot be accessed by the other side. That is, engram transfer does not occur.

Why should the commissures transfer sensory but not mnemonic information? By and large, commissural connections are homotopic, so that the fibers arise and terminate in the same general location but in opposite hemispheres (see Figure 7). A substantial proportion of the interhemispheric fibers arise and terminate in areas with specific sensory-perceptual functions. As a consequence, cross talk between these areas occurs. In contrast, mnemonic storage (as opposed to engram establishment) has not been successfully localized to specific cortical areas, and certain lines of evidence point to diffuse cortical and even subcortical involvement[26-29]. Thus, we feel that the specificity of the intrahemispheric cortical mechanisms involved could well account for the distinction between interhemispheric sensory and mnemonic transfer.

We are not suggesting, however, that commissural transmission is limited to sensory information. But the phylogenetic pervasiveness of sensory transfer does suggest that this form of interhemispheric communication may be the evolutionary model from which other types of transfer were derived. Moreover, the high proportion of interhemispheric fibers arising and terminating in brain areas with sensory-perceptual functions—in fish as well as in primates—further indicates that sensory transfer may be the prototype of interhemispheric communication in vertebrates.

Nevertheless, interhemispheric communication surely occurs

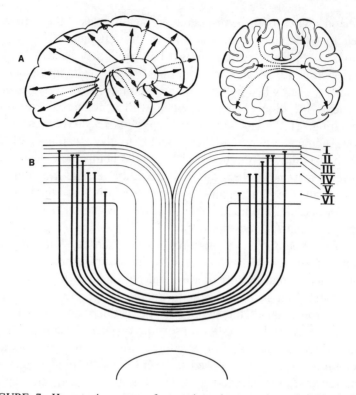

FIGURE 7. Homotopic nature of commissural connections. Interhemispheric fibers largely interconnect homologous areas in the two half-brains (Part A). In addition, they mostly terminate in the cortical laminae from which they arose in the opposite hemisphere (Part B).

between the motor and other cortical areas. Undoubtedly, as more is learned about neocortical organization, more clues concerning the nature of the commissural code will emerge. For example, there is some indication that learning-set formation (a conceptual task) involves the frontal cortex in monkeys[30], and indeed, Noble has demonstrated that when the frontal commissural connections are intact, both hemispheres acquire the concept[31]. Similarly, Gibson has shown that the anterior callosal connections may be critical for maintaining a motivational balance between the hemispheres[32].

Presumably, this effect is related to the anatomical relationship between the frontal cortex and the limbic system[33].

We are thus left with the view that the commissural system serves as a mechanism by which the neural activity—be it cognitive (sensory, perceptual, conceptual), conative (motivational, emotional), or motor activity—of highly specified cortical-cell populations in one half-brain is duplicated in the interrelated population in the opposite hemisphere. In the following section, we pursue the role of interhemispheric duplication, which really suggests why interhemispheric communication takes place.

The Role of Duplication

Why should nature go through all the trouble of providing a mechanism by which events occurring in one half-brain are duplicated in the other? The answer is actually quite simple; interhemispheric duplication provides for mental unity.

It is characteristic of bilateral nervous systems, which all vertebrates have, that sensory information concerning one half of space is isomorphically mapped onto one half-brain, while the other half-brain receives information concerning the other half of space. By way of interhemispheric communication, the lateralized maps are duplicated contralaterally. Each half-brain is thus provided with nearly simultaneous representations of both sensory spheres, and interhemispheric perceptual equilibrium is achieved. Therefore, we view interhemispheric communication as the mechanism by which the illusion of a single, complete psychological space is created from two separate neural representations of the same information (see Figure 8).

Perhaps there is no better way to grasp the critical role of interhemispheric cross-talk in the maintenance of psychological unity than to examine the subtle but real ways in which the mental life of the brain-bisected patient is "split" by commissurotomy. In the absence of the forebrain commissures, the patient's left hand no longer shares in the experiences of his right hand, and the visual world of each hemisphere is now totally contralateral[17]. Only

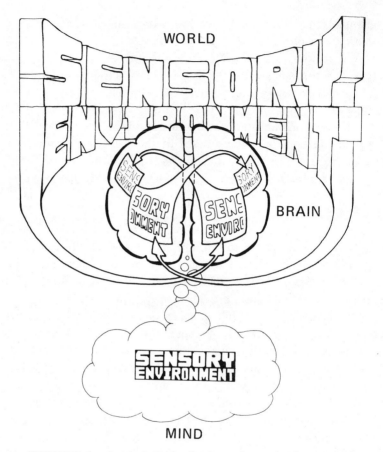

FIGURE 8. Interhemispheric duplication and mental unity (see text).

by continuous head and eye movements can the entirety of visual space be seen by both hemispheres. In addition, binocular depth perception is impaired[7]. Use of the left side of the body in a linguistic setting is limited[17], as are the manipulospatial abilities of the right side[34]. Moreover, bimanual motor coordination seems disturbed[90,91]. While we shall explore these and other distortions of consciousness throughout the remainder of the book, we need only realize here that just as a split brain produces a split mind, interhemispheric communication maintains mental unity.

WHERE? CLUES TO BASIC PRINCIPLES

Having specified what we feel is the nature of interhemispheric communication in terms of what transfers and why, we turn to the issue of where. Yet, coupled with the question of where information crosses between the hemispheres is the problem of how that information arrives at a hemisphere. That is, only when we are sure that the initial input is exclusively lateralized to one half-brain can we examine interhemispheric transfer.

We have chosen to focus on sensory transfer, with the goal being to uncover clues to basic principles of brain organization and function. We begin with a look at the variability and specificity that has been observed in the visual transfer mechanism, both within and between species. Our search for basic principles then continues within somatosensation, where the data prove consonant with an emerging theory concerning the central pathways for touch. The somatosensory system also provides the opportunity to explore the various psychological (ipsilateral cuing) and neurological (shifting circuits) strategies that surface to compensate for the loss of interhemispheric integration following commissurotomy.

VISUAL TRANSFER: VARIABILITY, SPECIFICITY, AND PLASTICITY IN BRAIN ORGANIZATION

The issue of where information transfers in the commissures is best analyzed in the visual system, where reports to date indicate a tremendous specificity of function. In addition, our clinical studies give the first clues as to the degree of variability that can exist in "where" information crosses in different individuals. Variability is also seen in the transfer mechanism of different groups of animals, with large differences occurring even in related species. With so much known about the visual transfer mechanism, it has served as a medium for examining neural plasticity and regenerative specificity. We will consider each of these points in turn.

The Human Anterior Commissure: Individual Differences in Visual Transfer

The anterior commissure has long been presumed to play a minor role in interhemispheric communication. This view, however, is undergoing a radical revision in light of our recent studies of interhemispheric transfer in patients with complete callosal sections but intact anterior commissures[16]. This prominent interhemispheric pathway interconnects various regions of the limbic cortex by way of the phylogenetically ancient anterior limb[35], which is found in all vertebrates[36], and also interconnects major portions of the neocortical temporal lobes by way of the posterior limb (Figure 9), which seems to be found only in primates[37-40]. Our main concern, for the present, is with those portions of the posterior limb that mediate interhemispheric visual communication between the visual areas of the temporal lobes.

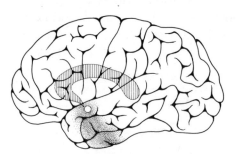

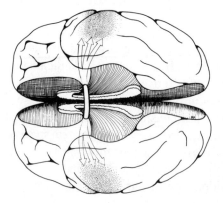

FIGURE 9. The anterior commissure in man. The approximate neocortical distribution of the posterior limb of the anterior commissure is shown. The superior aspect of the distribution is in the rostral part of the auditory-association cortex, while the inferior distribution is to the anterior part of the inferior temporal cortex, which is known from animal studies to play a critical role in visual processing.

Behavioral studies in nonhuman primates have clearly shown the anterior commissure to be capable of sustaining high-level interhemispheric visual communication[41−44]. In man, however, the situation is less clear-cut. While the anterior commissure clearly transfers visual information in some clinical cases, it clearly does not in others. We have recently observed five split-brain patients (D.H., P.S., J.Kn., D.S., and S.P.) who sustained complete sections of the corpus callosum with the anterior commissure left intact[16]. The extent of commissurotomy is shown in Figure 10. In four of these patients (D.H., J.Kn., D.S., and S.P.), the anterior commissure was found to be capable of transferring words, pictures of objects, and line drawings of nonsense figures. In the fifth, however, no transfer was seen.

The absence of transfer in P.S. is most readily accounted for by the fact that this patient suffered a unilateral temporal lesion at a very early age. This lesion may have disrupted or prevented the establishment of normal functional interhemispheric connections between the visual areas of the temporal lobes.

It is interesting to note that the observations made by Akelaitis in the 1940s were mainly on patients with callosum sections. The intact anterior commissure in these patients could clearly account, at least in part, for the fact that these patients failed to show the split-brain syndrome that was so dramatic in the Bogen and Vogel patients.

At the same time, the assumption that visual transfer through the anterior commissure is normally established during development is challenged by a number of scattered clinical reports. Surveys of the clinical literature have pointed out Maspes's[45] observation that section of the splenium (that part of the callosum containing the visual fibers in primates) results in the left hemisphere's being unable to read words and letters presented to the left visual field, yet these same patients could describe colors and objects in that field[46,47]. Treschner and Ford[48] described a similar case. Why is visual intercommunication disturbed at all in these patients with the anterior commissure intact?

Geschwind[49] has suggested that the anterior fiber pathways (including the rostral callosal fibers and the anterior commissure)

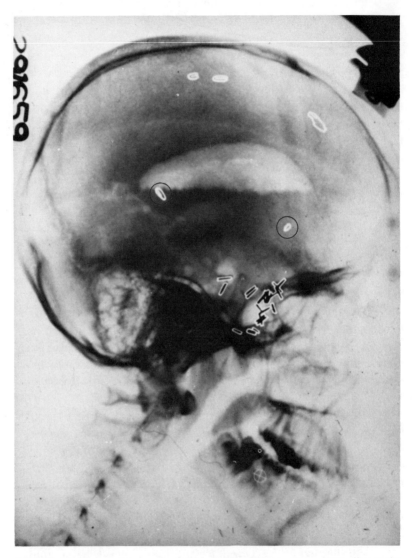

FIGURE 10. During the course of the surgery, Wilson places silver clips at the anterior and posterior borders of the callosal surgery, thereby allowing for post-operative X-ray verification of the extent of the section. The encircled clips are the ones of interest here.

may transfer some visual information but not complex visual symbols, such as words, citing as evidence the observation that splenial-lesioned patients with damage to the left occipital lobe do not manifest difficulty in naming objects. However, no disparity between the recognition of words as opposed to objects has been observed in our complete callosal-sectioned cases. Also, in a splenial-sectioned case recently reported, the patient was unable to report both words and pictures of objects[50].

One explanation for the inability of the anterior commissure to transfer visual information of a complex (i.e., verbal) nature in cases involving splenial lesions and left occipital damage, commonly referred to as *alexia without agraphia*, is that the alexia is not really attributable to inadequate interhemispheric integration via the anterior commissure but is instead due to poor intrahemispheric integration subsequent to successful transfer. Object naming, according to this interpretation, could be spared, as it might involve different patterns of circuitry than reading does.

Clearly, the anterior commissure has yet to reveal all of its secrets to us, particularly concerning the variability observed. Anatomically, it contains auditory[39] and olfactory[35] components, in addition to its visual fibers. Our behavioral data seem to correlate well with the anatomical picture, with the evidence for visual and olfactory transfer being the strongest[16]. As more patients with the anterior commissure intact become available, and as other clinical groups, such as alexics, are evaluated in light of these new observations, the story will undoubtedly unfold.

Comparative Variability in the Transfer Mechanism

The comparative approach to brain and behavior is currently enjoying an unprecedented wave of popularity among neurobiologists of various persuasions. As a consequence of this trend, it is becoming more and more apparent that an amazing degree of consistency characterizes the cerebral organization of the various vertebrates[51]. Studies of interhemispheric transfer certainly support this position, for fish, birds, and mammals have all been shown to exchange visual messages between their hemispheres[52]. However, this overwhelming emphasis on consistency has tended to obscure the diversity that exists in the visual transfer mechanism in various groups of vertebrates.

Interhemispheric communication is generally thought to take place by way of commissures—fiber tracts interconnecting brain areas at the same cerebral level—but in opposite hemispheres (i.e., between left and right visual cortices). This is certainly the case in mammals, where the forebrain commissures largely sustain cross-talk between the hemispheres. However, in nonmammals, interhemispheric visual communication takes place primarily by way of the supraoptic decussation[52]. Decussating fiber tracts are pathways that interconnect brain areas at different cerebral levels in opposite hemispheres (i.e., right tectum and left thalamus). In addition, however, it has recently been shown that under special training conditions, the tectal commissure can sustain a meaningful interhemispheric exchange of visual information in the fish[53].

Thus, in both mammals and nonmammals, sensory input from each visual field reaches both hemispheres, but the task is accomplished by quite distinct mechanisms in the different animal groups (see Figure 11). While transfer in mammals involves cortical–cortical processing between largely homologous brain areas, in nonmammals transfer occurs subcortically and generally involves nonhomologous areas at different cerebral levels, though

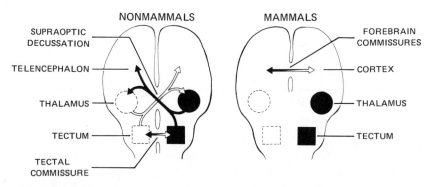

FIGURE 11. Transfer mechanisms in mammals and nonmammals. This figure shows schematically the functional neural circuitry involved in interhemispheric transfer in the different animals known to date.

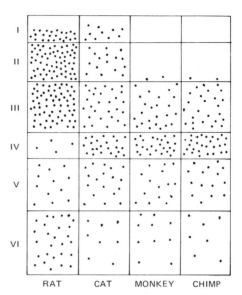

FIGURE 12. The unique laminar distribution of the commissural fibers in different mammals. Figure adapted from S. Jacobson and E. M. Marcus, 1969, Comparison of the laminar distribution of callosal synapses in the rat and rhesus monkey, *Anat. Rec. 163:*203.

homologous (tectal–tectal) transfer also occurs. The only evidence of any similarity at all in the transfer mechanism of mammals and nonmammals is Hamilton's observation that some low-level visual information may occasionally leak across the supraoptic decussation in the monkey[54].

Even within the mammals, interspecies variablity in the visual transfer mechanism abounds. Figure 12 depicts the huge differences seen in the terminal distribution of the forebrain commissures in the various cortical laminae of several mammals. To the extent that different cortical laminae are associated with different neural functions[36,55,56], interhemispheric communication may have unique adaptive significance in various creatures, above and beyond the basic transfer function.

Striking differences can also be found in the topographic organization of the visual commissures. In primates, the visual cortical areas of the occipital and temporal lobes send their interhemispheric fibers through the splenium of the corpus callosum and the anterior commissure[40]. This arrangement accounts for the observation that visual transfer can be mediated by either of these pathways in primates[16,41–44].

In the cat, since the anterior commissure does not interconnect cortical visual areas, it is not surprising that efforts to show visual transfer via this pathway have been unsuccessful[57]. What is surprising, however, is the observation that the splenium of the cat is only partially if at all involved in visual transfer. Myers found that sectioning of the anterior 87% of the callosum, which leaves a good part of the splenium intact, completely blocks visual transfer. Going in the other direction, he found that the posterior 45% of the callosum had to be cut to block transfer[58]. This finding indicates that visual transfer in the cat is mediated by callosal fibers mostly crossing the midline anterior to the splenium. This observation is consistent with the emerging cytoarchitectonic picture of the cat's visual cortex, which is now believed to include various extraoccipital cortical areas[59,60] that may well send their commissural axons anterior to the splenium (see Figure 13).

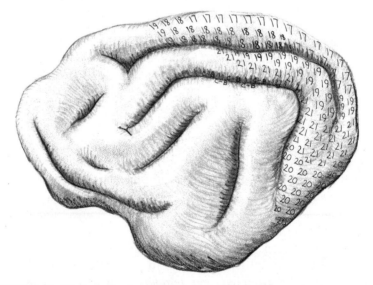

FIGURE 13. Cortical visual areas in the cat. The visual areas in the cat extend rostrally to an extent that suggests that the commissural axons may cross the midline rostral to the splenium. Figure adapted from C. J. Heath and E. G. Jones, 1971, The anatomical organization of the suprasylvian gyrus of the cat, *Erge. Anat. Entwicklungsgesch 45*:7–64.

While these huge differences in the visual transfer mechanism certainly do not negate the comparative approach, they nevertheless warn against wholesale interspecies generalizations. The same or similar function is accomplished by quite diverse mechanisms in different animals. Man is indeed not a fish or a cat. Keeping these cautions in mind, however, we turn to the fascinating issues of neural plasticity and specificity, which have been examined extensively in the fish and more recently, in the cat.

Neural Specificity

The continuing intrigue surrounding the degree and extent of neural specificity and the mechanisms of brain development remains as one of the truly central problems of neural science. Sperry's[61] brilliant work on the subject set up a framework for analysis, with every major neurobiologist working in the area trying to find a loophole in it. Yet, year after year, when the final analysis comes in, the extraordinary specificity of the nervous system that Sperry dramatically and somewhat counterintuitively proposed in the 1940s and 1950s continues to hold up.

Moving from that tradition, recent works by Andrew Francis and Lynn Bengston at Stony Brook have brought forth new evidence on the specificity of optic fibers' having to make connections in the tectum with second-order neurons that are involved in interhemispheric transfer[62]. In brief, goldfish that had had one optic nerve crushed and that were thus blind in one eye were allowed time for regeneration to take place. When vision returned, some were trained on a visual-pattern discrimination in the good eye and some initially in the regenerated eye. In both groups, excellent interocular transfer was seen, thereby showing that the specificity of new connections was great enough to make functional, correct connections with those neurons involved in relaying information over to the opposite half-brain.

Andrea Elberger has been studying the development of the callosum in the mammal with an eye on the question of the specificity of connections[63]. In an extraordinarily clever series of experiments, she first confirmed the findings of Anker and Cragg[64], showing that the splenial fibers do not develop across the midline to find their point of termination in the opposite hemisphere until the 22–72 postnatal day. This rather amazing fact may allow one the opportunity to block the natural path of these fibers during early development and to assess whether or not fibers found along a new path can specifically find the correct termination in the opposite half-brain. She has assessed the correct hookup behaviorally, by examining whether or not normal, binocular optic alignment is established. Elberger has shown that if section of the splenium is carried out early enough (13 days), optical alignment does not occur (see Figure 14).

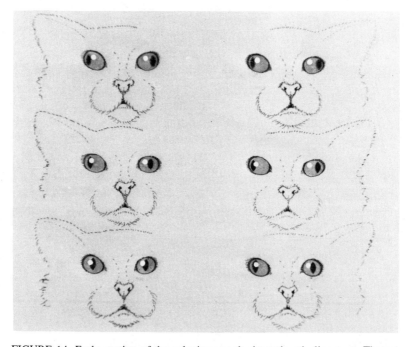

FIGURE 14. Early section of the splenium results in optic misalignment. The cat on the left is normal. The top illustration shows that when a single source of light (the white dot in each eye) is pointed at the normal kitten shortly after birth, the dot of light falls on different parts of the two eyes. Below this is the situation at six weeks. Finally, by the ninth week, the light falls on the same part of each eye, showing that optic alignment has been achieved. The kitten on the right is an example of what happens with early lesions of the splenium. In such cats, the eyes never align to the degree observed in normals.

What is of particular interest is the rather startling fact that splenial section in the adult cat does not impair optical alignment. This phenomenon would suggest that the neurological system crucial to the development of a particular sensorimotor function is not necessarily the one active in maintaining the function.

In the preceding, we spelled out some of the ways in which studies of the visual transfer mechanisms have begun to go beyond the basic issue of where information crosses. While the questions still outnumber the answers concerning the variability observed in the transfer capacity of the anterior commissure in human clinical cases, particularly between different patient populations, the animal studies described are suggestive of some truly exciting mechanisms and, moreover, some new approaches to old but persistent questions. The comparative variability observed in the transfer mechanism is important to keep in mind, for it warns us about being too complacent in attributing similar behavioral functions in different species to identical neural mechanisms.

LATERALITY EFFECTS IN SOMESTHESIS: CLUES TO SOMATOSENSORY ORGANIZATION, CUING STRATEGIES, AND SHIFTING CIRCUITS

The problem of measuring interhemispheric communication is always complicated by the ever-present difficulty in first being certain that the stimulus information is lateralized to one half-brain. It has long been assumed that one could achieve this by simply localizing somatosensory input to one side of the body, for it was generally believed that the cerebral projection of the various somatic afferents was largely contralateral for all parts of the body except the head and neck. Yet, studies of split-brain animals and humans have suggested a surprising degree of homolateral somatosensory representation, which raises the question of whether it is possible to truly lateralize somatosensory input. As it turns out, when the two major ascending somatosensory pathways are considered separately in terms of their known anatomical, physiological, and behavior properties, a model of laterality effects in somesthesis does indeed emerge.

Somatosensory Organization

The somatosensory system is multimodal, containing touch, temperature, proprioceptive, pain, and other components. These various modalities are mediated by two ascending pathways: the dorsal-column–medial-lemniscal system and the spinothalamic system. For quite some time, the dorsal-column–lemniscal system was thought to be the pathway for discrete touch (stereognosis, feature identification, tactile localization, etc.), with the spinothalamic handling other, less discrete forms of touch sensitivity, as well as pain and temperature[65].

In recent years, a new view of somatosensory organization, regarding the pathways for touch, has emerged[66–70]. The dorsal-column–lemniscal system seems to be more involved in active touch[71] than in the mediation of discrete touch per se. Complete dorsal-column transsection eliminates the capacity for learning tactual discriminations that require active exploration of the stimulus features. In contrast, passive touch, which is sufficient for discriminations that have a single key dimension upon which correct performance is dependent (such as roughness, texture, form, and localization discriminations), survives dorsal-column lesions.

The foregoing observations, in conjunction with the classical notions concerning pain and temperature[65], suggest that the dorsal-column–medial-lemniscal system is the pathway for active touch and proprioception and that passive touch, pain, and temperature sensations are transmitted centrally by way of the spinothalamic system. Consider the anatomical organization of these two pathways.

The dorsal-column–medial-lemniscal pathway is completely crossed, connecting various points on the body with the opposite half-brain (see Figure 15A). The thalamic termination of this system is in the nucleus VPL, which contains only contralateral cells[72]. On the other hand, the spinothalamic system terminates in VPL and the posterior thalamus contralaterally, but also in the homolateral posterior thalamus[72]. The homolateral projection is not an ipsilateral projection per se but instead seems to be by way of doubly decussating fibers that recross the midline in the brain stem[73], as shown in Figure 15B.

Thus, while the dorsal-column–lemniscal pathway is a contralateral system, the spinothalamic projection has homolateral and contralateral components. Therefore, one should expect to find crisp lateralization of dorsal-column information (active touch, proprioception) but various degrees of lateralization for information transmitted centrally by way of the spinothalamic system (passive touch, pain, temperature). Studies of brain-bisected subjects wholly support this model.

Human Studies

One of the first problems systematically attacked in the California patients was that of somesthesis. Three patients were tested on a variety of somesthetic tasks, including proprioceptive, stereognostic, thermal, and pain discriminations, as well as tactual localization[74,75].

Proprioception. In tests of joint and position sensation, the various joints—such as the wrist, shoulder, elbow, knee, and ankle—were placed in given positions by the examiner; then the subject, wearing a blindfold, was required to state verbally the position of the relevant distal portion of the limb. The task presented no problem for the right hand and foot, but proved difficult when the description involved the joint position of the left wrist, the left fingers, and the left toes. Sense of position at the left shoulder and probably also at the left elbow was preserved. Position was correctly reported without difficulty for all joints on the right arm and also for the left knee and ankle. When the right arm was held out simultaneously with the left, however, thereby equalizing and obscuring the secondary mechanical tensions across the spinal column, ability to describe the position of the left arm dropped to chance. Also, when the end of a pencil was held in one hand and positioned by the experimenter at different angles and positions, the subject was unable to reach accurately for the other end of the pencil with the opposite hand. Taken together, these observations suggest that proprioception is crisply lateralized.

Tactual Localization. The patients were required to localize, either verbally or by pointing, the spot on the skin at which a brief tactual stimulus was applied. Throughout all phases of testing, the

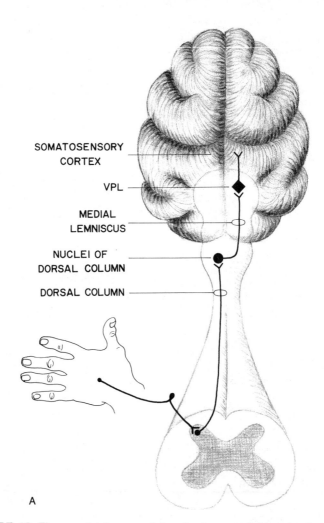

SOMATOSENSORY
CORTEX

VPL

MEDIAL
LEMNISCUS

NUCLEI OF
DORSAL COLUMN

DORSAL COLUMN

A

FIGURE 15. The completely crossed dorsal-column-medial-lemniscal system is shown in Part A. Part B depicts the spinothalamic system, which has crossed and uncrossed components. The uncrossed component, however, is really a doubly decussating component that allows somatosensory information from one side of the body to reach the ipsilateral half-brain.

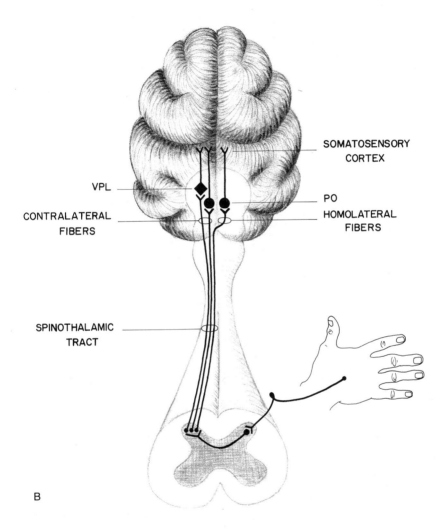

<table>
</table>

SOMATOSENSORY
CORTEX

VPL

PO

CONTRALATERAL
FIBERS

HOMOLATERAL
FIBERS

SPINOTHALAMIC
TRACT

B

patients were able to accurately localize cutaneous stimulation on either side of the face and on the top and the back of the head.

Below the neck, as long as the stimulus and the response were on the same side of the body, the patients were able to identify the point of stimulation. When the patient was required to find a point on one side of the body using the opposite hand, performance broke down. Similarly, verbal descriptions of the point of stimulation were accurate for points on the right side of the body but not for points on the left. With increasing postoperative time, however, there was a dramatic improvement in cross-localization facility for all body points, except the hands, in two patients. The greater degree of extracallosal brain damage in the third patient probably accounted for his failure to acquire cross-localization skills for points on the torso and the proximal extremities.

Stereognosis. In psychological tests of stereognosis, intermanual transfer of tactile discriminations was generally not seen. On the average, tactile-memory problems in which the patients learned to choose one of two stimuli on one trial showed no transfer. Test objects placed in one hand could easily be retrieved with the same hand, but not with the opposite hand, from a grab bag containing 10 objects. Yet, the patients were able to identify verbally certain diffuse features of objects in the left hand, such as curvature, edges, weight, and the like.

Clearly, since the patients with more-or-less pure commissural lesions were able to report a considerable amount about the nature of left-sided stimulation, it seemed likely that some simple object held in the left hand might be correctly named by the patients. This proved to be the case. If only two objects were available for palpation, such as a round ball and a square, and the subject was informed that only these two stimuli would be used, the two cases with pure lesions performed at a high level when asked to call out which of the two had been placed in the left hand. If these same two objects were presented in series with a number of other objects and no "verbal set" was given limiting what might be presented, a poor score resulted.

Thus, it came to be seen that this kind of ipsilateral cuing mechanism allows leakage of some types of information about the nature of objects held in one hand over to the ipsilateral hemisphere. It works much more efficiently if the receiving brain is "set" and the conditions for response are limited. We will examine ipsilateral cuing in more detail when we consider the animal studies.

Temperature and Pain. It is generally believed that pain and temperature sensations on one side of the body reach both cerebral hemispheres, and by the same central pathways[65]. As it turned out, crossed discriminations could be made for both pain[75] and temperature[76].

Conclusions. These observations on brain-bisected humans are consistent with and lend credence to the model of somatosensation put forward. The dorsal columns, which are completely crossed, mediate proprioception. Thus, the joint and position senses are crisply lateralized. In contrast, the passive touch functions mediated by the spinothalamic pathways show various degrees of bilateral representation. While it is clear that the contralateral representation of stereognostic and tactual localization skills exceeds the ipsilateral representation, in the case of pain and temperature sensations complete bilateral representation is the rule.

Before we leave this topic, it is important to point out the extent to which intermanual cross-talk improved in the postoperative months on both the stereognostic and the localization tasks. While these observations can be accounted for in part by behavioral compensation strategies (see the section on "Animal Studies"), there is also some indication that the capacity of the homolateral spinothalamic pathways increases following commissurotomy.

One way of looking at these "shifting circuits" is that diffuse ipsilateral representation is not needed, given a functioning callosal system. Both hemispheres are kept current as to the status of both sides of the body by way of interhemispheric transmission. Once the commissural sensory window is lost, however, the only source of ipsilateral information is by way of the homolateral spinothalamic projections. That these pathways are not available immediately following commissurotomy suggests that while they are physiologically active[72], they become functionally useful only when a real need is established.

For example, hemispherectomized animals manifest dramatic sensorimotor losses immediately after surgery, but the intact hemisphere gains more and more control over the homolateral body during the postoperative period. Similarly, observations of hemispherectomized humans suggest that potential homolateral pathways may lie dormant or undeveloped in the normal brain[77,78].

Our own observations of case J.H. are also indicative of shifting somatosensory circuits. Following complete forebrain commissurotomy, severe medical complications set in, and recovery was slow for J.H. Although his left hemisphere could respond appropriately to right-visual-field and right-hand stimulations, his right hemisphere generally failed to respond at all. Throughout the postoperative period, however, we have seen a gradual but consistent increase in J.H.'s ability to respond to left-hand information with his left hemisphere. This increase suggests that the extensive damage to his right hemisphere, due to his presurgical pathology as well as to postsurgical complications, created a real need for ipsilateral representation of the left hand in the left hemisphere. With time, this need seems to have been met.

Animal Studies

A variety of studies of somesthesis in split-brain animals have been conducted. In general, these studies have focused on form discriminations, texture discriminations, and latch-box learning. While form and texture discriminations merely require passive touch, latch-box learning requires the active exploration of a multidimensional stimulus situation. Consequently, in callosal-sectioned animals, we might expect to find little evidence of intermanual transfer of latch-box learning but perhaps some leakage of form and texture information.

Myers[79] and Semmes and Mishkin[80] reported no evidence for intermanual transfer of form and texture information in split-brain monkeys. However, Sperry[81] and Ettlinger and Morton[82] found excellent transfer of form and texture in callosum-sectioned monkeys. Although Glickstein and Sperry[83] concluded that callosal sectioning interferes with and may completely block the transfer of somesthetic information in monkeys, their data indicate that form and texture information "leaked" across the midline on 4 of 12 tests. In addition, Stamm and Sperry[84] also concluded that callosal section blocks intermanual transfer of form and texture, but they reported on one split cat with a substantial savings. In contrast to these variable results for form and texture discriminations, Henson and Myers[85] and Kohn and Myers[86] found no evidence for a savings in relearning of latch-box problems by the untrained hand in primates. Thus, only passive touch seems to leak across in splits, and only occasionally.

Ipsilateral Cuing. In a split-brain animal, the contralateral hemisphere alone receives the dorsal-column information necessary for active touch. Thus, the untrained hemisphere remains essentially naive on latch-box problems. However, as we have seen, some information from the passive touch (spinothalamic) system reaches both hemispheres. Although primary stereognostic information is available only to the contralateral hemisphere, such secondary dimensions as weight, number of edges, the presence or absence of stimulation, and the like are diffuse stimulus aspects that can be homolaterally identified[87]. While these features are sometimes the relevant dimension in discrete passive-touch situations, in cases where they are not, they can frequently be used to distinguish the discriminanda, if only on a primitive level.

It is interesting that although cats have more bilateral representation than primates[88], there is more evidence for intermanual transfer in split-brain monkeys. This difference is understandable if we assume that ipsilateral cuing depends to some extent on the creativity of the individual animal (as well as on the complexity of the test situation). Because monkeys are likely to be more ingenious than cats, there is more evidence for transfer in split monkeys.

One mechanism by which cuing might take place requires that the untrained hemisphere store the secondary cues available during original training. When tested, the untrained hemisphere merely matches the secondary cues of the test situation with those acquired during training and then responds appropriately. Another possibility is that the trained hemisphere matches diffuse secondary cues available during testing with its store of secondary cues from training. On this basis, the trained hemisphere could either initiate the response itself (as long as the response does not require precise finger movements, which are under exclusive contralateral control) or could signal (by face movements, body tilt, or some other peripheral cue) to the untrained hemisphere when to respond. This latter cuing strategy is called *cross-cuing* and has been considered in detail elsewhere[17,87].

These notions are supported by studies showing that cuing in split subjects can be eliminated if such compensation strategies are made difficult to carry out. For example, Lee-Teng and Sperry[89] have shown that if an intermanual paired-comparison task is made more complex by an increase in the number of comparison possibilities, intermanual transfer is eliminated.

Thus, cuing is commonly seen in passive touch situations because the spinothalamic system can frequently hand information sufficient to mediate correct responding, although the information is secondary to tactual gnosis per se. These mechanisms, which are to some extent dependent on the ingenuity of the individual animal and the specific aspects of the test situation, explain the variability in the passive touch literature. Furthermore, cuing strategies are not seen in situations requiring active exploration (e.g., latch-box problems) because the complex, multidimensional nature of such situations precludes the simple identification of the appropriate stimulus features and because there are no homolateral fibers that can convey the necessary information (proprioceptive feedback from active palpation) to the responding hemisphere.

So, we can see that when the topic of laterality effects in somesthesis is approached with a clear understanding of the structural and functional properties of the distinct somatic afferent pathways, the data seem to make good sense. Those functions (active touch, proprioception) clearly mediated by the crossed dorsal-column–lemniscal system are well lateralized. In contrast, because the spinothalamic system has both crossed and homolateral components, its functions (passive touch, pain, and temperature) show various degrees of bilateral representation. Furthermore, it is interesting to note the neurological (shifting circuits) and psychological (ipsilateral cuing) strategies that emerge following commissurotomy to offset the breakdown in the flow of somatosensory information between the hemispheres. It is as if the brain demands integration, and in the absence of the interhemispheric pathways, less efficient ways of achieving mental unity are employed. As we will see in the final chapter, a very powerful mechanism of the mind is revealed by observations of how the verbal system of the split-brain patient attempts to reintegrate the conscious processes that have been fragmented by commissurotomy.

CONCLUSION

We began this chapter with a theoretical issue: What is it that is transferred between the hemispheres, and why does it transfer? Basically, we believe that the interhemispheric pathways transfer highly specified neural codes that serve to maintain an informational balance across the cerebral midline, and in doing so, provide for mental unity.

Once one accepts such a view of commissural function, it becomes difficult to work with the two-brain model of normal cerebral organization that has evolved out of the split-brain work. Instead, it becomes more attractive to view the hemispheres as intimately associated and working in synchrony. So, in the next chapter, our goal is to critically examine the two-brain model, which is to say, the theory of hemisphere specialization.

REFERENCES

1. D. H. Hubel and T. N. Wiesel, 1962, Receptive fields, binocular interaction and functional architecture in the cat's visual cortex, *J. Physiol. (London)* *160*:106–154.
2. D. H. Hubel and T. N. Wiesel, 1967, Cortical and callosal connections concerned with the vertical meridian of visual fields in the cat, *J. Neurophysiol.* *30*:1561–1573.
3. B. P. Choudhury, D. Whitteridge, and M. E. Wilson. 1965. The function of

the callosal connections of the visual cortex, *Quart. J. Exp. Physiol.* *50:*214–219.

4. G. Berlucchi and G. Rizzolatti, 1968, Binocularly driven neurons in visual cortex of split-chiasm cats, *Science 159:*308.

5. G. Berlucchi, M. S. Gazzaniga, and G. Rizzolatti, 1967, Microelectrode analysis of transfer of visual information by the corpus callosum of cat, *Arch. Ital. Biol. 105:*583–596.

6. C. Blakemore, 1970, Binocular depth perception and the optic chiasm, *Vision Res. 10:*43–47.

7. D. Mitchell and C. Blakemore, 1969, Binocular depth perception and the corpus callosum, *Vision Res. 10:*49–54.

8. C. E. Rocha-Miranda, D. B. Bender, C. G. Gross, and M. Mishkin, 1975, Visual activation of neurons in inferotemporal cortex depends on striate cortex and forebrain commissures, *J. Neurophysiol. 38:*475–491.

9. R. E. Myers, 1955, Interocular transfer of pattern discrimination in cats following section of crossed optic fibers, *J. Comp. Physiol. Psychol. 48:*470–473.

10. R. E. Myers, 1961, Corpus callosum and visual gnosis, in: A. Fessard, R. W. Gerard, J. Konorski, and J. F. Delafresnaye (Eds.), *Brain Mechanism and Learning,* Oxford, Blackwell Scientific Publications, p. 481.

11. R. E. Myers, 1962, Transmission of visual information within and between the hemispheres: a behavioral study, in: V. B. Mountcastle, (Ed.), *Interhemispheric Relations and Cerebral Dominance,* Baltimore, The Johns Hopkins Press, pp. 51–73.

12. R. E. Myers, 1965, The neocortical commissures and interhemispheric transmission of information, in: E. G. Ettlinger (Ed.), *Functions of the Corpus Callosum,* London, J. A. Churchill, pp. 1–17.

13. R. W. Doty, N. Negrao, and K. Yamaga, 1973, The unilateral engram, *Acta Neurobiol. Exp. 33:*711–728.

14. C. R. Butler, 1968, A memory-record for visual discrimination habits produced in both cerebral hemispheres of monkey when only one hemisphere has received direct visual information, *Brain Res. 10:*152–167.

15. C. R. Hamilton, 1976, Investigations of perceptual and mnemonic lateralization in monkeys, in: S. Harnad (Ed.), *Lateralization in the Nervous System,* New York, Academic Press.

16. G. L. Risse, J. LeDoux, D. H. Wilson, and M. S. Gazzaniga, 1977, Role of anterior commissure in interhemispheric transfer in man, *Neuropsychologia,* in press.

17. M. S. Gazzaniga, 1970, *The Bisected Brain,* New York, Appleton-Century-Crofts.

18. J. W. Kling and L. A. Riggs, 1971, *Experimental Psychology* (3rd ed.), New York, Holt, Rinehart, Winston.

19. C. E. Rocha-Miranda, D. B. Bender, C. G. Gross, and M. Mishkin, 1975,

Visual activation of neurons in inferotemporal cortex depends on striate cortex and forebrain commissures, *J. Neurophysiol. 38:*475–491.

20. R. E. Myers and R. W. Sperry, 1953, Interocular transfer of a visual form discrimination habit in cats after section of the optic chiasm and corpus callosum, *Anat. Rec. 175:*351–352.

21. I. S. Russell and S. Ochs, 1961, One-trial interhemispheric transfer of a learning engram, *Science 133:*1077–1078.

22. T. J. Carew, T. J. Crow, and L. Petrinovich, 1970, Lack of coincidence between neural and behavioral manifestations of cortical spreading depression, *Science 169:*1339–1342.

23. I. S. Russell, 1971, Neurological basis of complex learning, *Br. Med. Bull. 27:*278–285.

24. L. Petrinovich, 1976, Cortical spreading depression and memory transfer: A methodological critique, *Behav. Biol. 16:*79.

25. G. L. Risse and M. S. Gazzaniga, 1976, Verbal retrieval of right hemisphere memories established in the absence of language, *Neurology 26:*354.

26. K. S. Lashley, 1950, In search of the engram, *Symposia of the Society for Experimental Biology 4:*454–482.

27. R. Thompson and R. E. Myers, 1971, Brainstem mechanisms underlying visually guided responses in the rhesus monkey, *J. Comp. Physiol. Psychol. 74:*479–512.

28. R. Thompson, 1965, Centrencephalic theory and interhemispheric transfer of visual habits, *Psychol. Rev.* 72(5)385–398.

29. R. Thompson, 1961, Localization of the "visual memory system" in the white rat, *J. Comp. Physiol. Psychol.* 69(4)1–29.

30. M. Mishkin, 1969, Perseveration of central sets after frontal lesions in monkeys, in: J. M. Warren and K. Akert (Eds.), *The Frontal Granular Cortex and Behaviour,* New York, McGraw-Hill, pp. 219–241.

31. J. Noble, 1973, Interocular transfer in the monkey; rostral corpus callosum mediates transfer of object learning set but not of single-problem learning, *Brain Res. 50:*147–162.

32. A. Gibson and M. S. Gazzaniga, 1971, Differences in eating behavior in split-brain monkeys, *Physiologist 14:*50.

33. W. J. H. Nauta, 1969, Some efferent connections of the prefrontal cortex in the monkey, in: J. M. Warren and K. Akert (Eds.), *The Frontal Granular Cortex and Behavior,* New York, McGraw-Hill, pp. 397–409.

34. J. LeDoux, D. H. Wilson, and M. S. Gazzaniga, 1977, Manipulospatial aspects of cerebral lateralization: Clues to the origin of lateralization, *Neuropsychologia,* in press.

35. C. A. Fox and J. T. Schmitz, 1943, A Marchi study of the distribution of the anterior commissure in the cat, *J. Comp. Neurol. 89:*297–304.

36. E. C. Crosby, T. Humphrey, and E. W. Lauer, 1962, *Correlative Anatomy of the Nervous System,* New York, Macmillan.

37. D. G. Whitlock and W. J. H. Nauta, 1956, Subcortical projections from temporal neocortex in *Macaca mulatta, J. Comp. Neurol. 106:*183–212.
38. J. Klinger and P. Gloor, 1960, The connections of amygdala and the anterior temporal cortex in the human brain, *J. Comp. Neurol. 115:*333–369.
39. D. N. Pandya, M. Hallett, and S. K. Mukherjee, 1969, Intra- and interhemispheric connections of the neocortical auditory systems in the rhesus monkey, *Brain Res. 14:*49–65.
40. S. M. Zeki, 1973, Comparison of the cortical degeneration in the visual region of temporal lobe of the monkey following section of the anterior commissure and the splenium, *J. Comp. Neurol. 143:*167–175.
41. P. Black and R. E. Myers, 1965, Visual function of the forebrain commissures in the chimpanzee, *Science 146:*799.
42. M. S. Gazzaniga, 1966, Interhemispheric communication of visual learning, *Neuropsychologia 4:*183–189.
43. M. V. Sullivan and C. R. Hamilton, 1973, Interocular transfer of reversed and nonreversed discriminations via the anterior commissure in monkeys, *Physiol. Behav. 10:*355–359.
44. R. W. Doty and W. H. Overman, 1976, Mnemonic role of forebrain commissures in Macaques, in: S. Harnad (Ed.), *Lateralization in the nervous system,* New York, Academic Press.
45. P. E. Maspes, 1948, Le syndrôme experimental chez l'homme de la section du splenium du corps calleux, *Alexie Visuelle Pure Hemianopsique Rev. 80:*100–113.
46. F. Bremer, J. Brihaye, and G. Andre-Balisaux, 1956, Physiologie et pathologie du corps calleux, *Arch. Suisses Neurol. Psychiatr. 48:*411–414.
47. N. Geschwind, 1965, Disconnection syndrome in animals and man, *Brain 88:*237–294.
48. J. H. Treschner and R. F. Ford, 1937, Colloid cyst of the third ventricle, *Arch. Neurol. Psychiatr. (Chic.) 37:*959–973.
49. N. Geschwind, 1974, Discussion, in: F. Michel and B. Schott (Eds.), *Les syndrômes de disconnexion calleuse chez l'homme,* Lyon, France, Colloque International de Lyon.
50. M. S. Gazzaniga and H. Freedman, 1973, Observations on visual processes after posterior callosal section, *Neurology 23:*1126–1130.
51. W. J. H. Nauta and H. Karten, 1970, A general profile of the vertebrate brain, with sidelights on the ancestry of cerebral cortex, *The Neurosciences: Second Study Program,* New York, Rockefeller University Press.
52. M. Cuénod, 1972, Split-brain studies: Functional interaction between bilateral central nervous structures, in: G. Bourne (Ed.), *Structure and Function of Nervous Tissue,* New York, Academic Press, Vol. 5, pp. 445–504.
53. C. L. Bengston, A. Francis, and M. S. Gazzaniga, 1977, Interocular transfer tests following tectal commissure section in goldfish, in preparation.
54. C. R. Hamilton, personal communication.
55. M. A. Jacobson and H. Hirsch, 1975, The perfectible brain: Principles of

neuronal development, in: M. S. Gazzaniga and C. Blakemore (Eds.), *Handbook of Psychobiology*, New York, Academic Press.

56. D. H. Hubel, and T. N. Wiesel, Receptive fields, binocular interaction and functional architecture in the cat's visual cortex, *J. Physiol. (London) 160:*106–154.

57. C. R. Hamilton, personal communication.

58. R. E. Myers, 1956, Localization of function within the corpus callosum, *Anat. Rec. 124:*339.

59. C. J. Heath and E. G. Jones, 1970, Connections of area in and lateral suprasylvian area of cat's visual cortex, *Brain Res. 19:*302–305.

60. D. H. Hubel and T. N. Wiesel, 1969, Visual areas of the lateral suprasylvian cortex of the cat, *J. Physiol. (London) 202:*251–260.

61. R. W. Sperry, 1948, Patterning of central synapses in regeneration of optic nerve in teleosts, *Physiol. Zool. 21:*351–361.

62. A., Francis, L. O. Bengston, and M. S. Gazzaniga, 1976, Interocular equivalence after optic nerve regeneration in goldfish, *Exp. Neurol. 53:*94–101.

63. A. Elberger, 1977, Behavioral and anatomical results of posterior callosal section in neonatal cats, unpublished doctoral thesis, SUNY at Stony Brook, New York.

64. R. Anker and B. Cragg, 1974, The development of the extrinsic connections of the visual cortex in the cat, *J. Comp. Neurol. 154:*29–41.

65. V. B. Mountcastle and I. Darien-Smith, 1968, Neural mechanisms in somesthesia, in: V. B. Mountcastle (Ed.), *Medical Physiology*, St. Louis, Mosby Press.

66. J. Semmes and M. Mishkin, 1965, Somatosensory loss in monkeys after ipsilateral cortical ablation, *J. Neurophysiol. 28:*473–486.

67. R. J. Schwartzman and J. Semmes, 1971, The sensory cortex and tactile sensitivity, *Exp. Neurol. 37:*147–158.

68. P. D. Wall, 1970, The sensory and motor role of impulses travelling in the dorsal columns toward cerebral cortex, *Brain 93:*505–524.

69. P. D. Wall, 1975, The somatosensory system, in: M. S. Gazzaniga (Ed.), *Handbook of Psychobiology*, New York, Academic Press.

70. A. Azulay and A. S. Schwartz, 1975, The role of the dorsal funiculus of the primate in tactile discrimination, *Exp. Neurol. 46:*315–332.

71. J. J. Gibson, 1962, Observations on active touch, *Psychol. Rev. 69:*477–491.

72. G. F. Poggio and V. B. Mountcastle, 1960, A study of the functional contribution of the lemniscal and spinothalamic systems to somatic sensibility, *Bull. Johns Hopkins Hosp. 106:*266–316.

73. F. W. L. Kerr, 1975, The ventral spinothalamic tract and other ascending systems of the ventral funiculus of the spinal cord, *J. Comp. Neurol. 159:*335–356.

74. M. S. Gazzaniga, J. E. Bogen, and R. W. Sperry, 1963, Laterality effects in somesthesis following cerebral commissurotomy in man, *Neuropsychologia 1:*209–215.

75. M. S. Gazzaniga, 1965, Some effects of cerebral commissurotomy in monkey and man, *Diss. Abstr. 26:*1.

76. J. Levy and R. W. Sperry, 1970, Crossed temperature discrimination following section of forebrain neocortical commissures, *Cortex 6:*349–361.

77. W. J. Gardner, L. J. Karnosh, J. R. McClure, C. Christopher, and A. K. Gardner, 1955, Residual function following hemispherectomy for tumour and for infantile hemiplegia, *Brain 78:*487.

78. R. H. White, L. H. Schreiner, R. A. Hughes, C. S. MacCarty, and J. H. Gridlay, 1959, Physiological consequences of total hemispherectomy in the monkey: Operative method and functional recovery, *Neurology (Minneap.) 6:*149.

79. R. E. Myers, 1965, The neocortical commissures and interhemispheric transmission of information, in: E. G. Ettlinger (Ed.), *Functions of the Corpus Callosum,* London, J. A. Churchill, pp. 1–17.

80. J. Semmes and M. Mishkin, 1965, Somatosensory loss in monkeys after ipsilateral cortical ablation, *J. Neurophysiol. 28:*473–486.

81. R. W. Sperry, 1958, The corpus callosum and interhemispheric transfer in the monkey, *Anat. Rec. 131:*297.

82. G. Ettlinger and H. B. Morton, 1966, Tactile discrimination performance in the monkey; Transfer of training between the hands after commissural section, *Cortex 2:*30–49.

83. M. Glickstein and R. W. Sperry, 1960, Intermanual somesthetic transfer in split-brain rhesus monkey, *J. Comp. Physiol. Psychol. 53:*322.

84. J. S. Stamm and R. W. Sperry, 1957, Function of corpus callosum in contralateral transfer of somesthetic discrimination in cats, *J. Comp. Physiol. Psychol. 50:*138.

85. R. E. Myers and C. O. Henson, 1960, Role of corpus callosum in transfer of tactuokinesthetic learning in chimpanzees, *Arch. Neurol. 3:*404–409.

86. B. Kohn and R. E. Myers, 1969, Visual information and intermanual transfer of latch box problem solving in monkeys with commissures sectioned, *Exp. Neurol. 23:*303–309.

87. M. S. Gazzaniga, 1969, Cross cuing mechanisms and ipsilateral eye-hand control in split-brain monkeys, *Exp. Neurol. 23:*11–17.

88. J. E. Rose and V. B. Mountcastle, 1960, Touch and kinesthesis, in: J. Field, H. W. Magoun, and V. E. Hall (Eds.), *Handbook of Physiology: Neurophysiology, II,* Washington, American Physiological Society.

89. E. Lee-Teng and R. W. Sperry, 1966, Intermanual stereognostic size discrimination in split-brain monkeys, *J. Comp. Physiol. Psychol. 62:*84–89.

90. B. F. B. Preilowski, 1972, Possible contribution of the anterior forebrain commissures to bilateral motor coordination, *Neuropsychologia 10:*256–277.

91. D. Zaidel and R. W. Sperry, 1977, Long-term motor coordination problems following cerebral commissurotomy in man, *Neuropsychologia 15:*193–204.

3

Cerebral Lateralization and Hemisphere Specialization
Facts and Theory

The human brain seems mysteriously unique in phylogeny. In addition to being unpredictably large, man's brain differs from its anthropoid legacy in that the two halves are functionally asymmetric, with the left performing better on verbal tasks and the right excelling in some situations demanding nonverbal skills. These observations have led to the view that each half-brain has evolved its own specialized neural substrate to sustain a unique cognitive style and mode of information processing.

We feel that this popular view of lateralization goes well beyond the data from which it emerged. It is thus our goal in this chapter first to clarify what the facts concerning lateralization are and then to spell out in more detail the inferences that have surfaced to explain lateralized processes. Given this overview, we go on to describe our recent experiments that have suggested a simple but viable theory of the origins of cerebral lateralization. The theory is appealing in that it places the human brain on a neuro-evolutionary continuum with its primate ancestry.

CEREBRAL LATERALIZATION: THE FACTS

The clinical observations of Broca, Wernicke, and other 19th-century neurologists provided the first clues concerning the lateralization of function in the human brain. The high correlation between aphasic disorders and left-hemisphere lesions in right-handed persons suggested that the neural substrate of language was primarily localized to the left half of the neocortical mass, which came to be referred to as the major or dominant hemisphere. In contrast, the right hemisphere was relegated to a minor or nondominant position because of the conspicuous absence of evidence that this half-brain played other than a minimal role in higher cortical function, except for Hughlings Jackson's speculation that the right hemisphere might be critically involved in visual ideation[1].

By the mid-20th century, however, it was obvious that the major–minor partition of cerebral functioning applied only to linguistic mechanisms and not to the overall pattern of cerebral activity. As early as 1935, Weisenburg and McBride had reported that patients with right-hemisphere lesions, unlike those with left lesions, performed poorly on tests involving the manipulation and appreciation of forms and spatial relationships[2], with a host of subsequent clinical studies confirming the disruptive effects of right-hemisphere lesions on spatial functions[3-17]. In addition, right-hemisphere lesions were found to produce greater deficits than left lesions on tests of visual and auditory perception, as well as on tests of visual memory[18-24]. Similarly, studies of hemisphere function in normal subjects revealed a right-hemisphere advantage on some visual and auditory perceptual tasks.[25,26,69,72,79,80]

The emergence of the Bogen and Vogel[27] series of split-brain patients added new dimensions to the study of hemisphere function. Each hemisphere could be studied independently of the contaminating effects of the other half-brain, and hemisphere function could be assessed directly rather than by the inferring of function from the capacities lost following damage to one or the other hemisphere.

The initial studies of Gazzaniga, Bogen, and Sperry[28-32] confirmed in dramatic fashion the conclusions drawn from the earlier studies of clinical and normal subjects, and later studies of the same patients using a variety of tasks extended the initial findings[33-39]. In general, the left hemisphere was found to excel in situations demanding verbal processing, while the right performed in a superior fashion on tasks requiring nonverbal skills.

HEMISPHERE SPECIALIZATION

The studies of normal, brain-lesioned, and split-brain subjects have all led to the same conclusion: in man, each hemisphere is endowed with certain capacities that are either lacking or poorly represented in the other half-brain. Such are the facts of cerebral lateralization. From these facts, inferences concerning the unitary nature of hemisphere function have emerged. The hemispheres have come to be viewed as possessing unique, evolved cognitive styles, and various dichotomies have been offered to contrast the distinct modes[40].

The current and generally accepted model of unitary hemisphere function is that of cerebral specialization. Unfortunately, the facts of lateralization have merged with the inferences. Lateralization has come to imply specialization.

Specialization theory assumes that the phylogenetic emergence of the human brain was associated with, and even dependent upon, the radical reorganization of cerebral function, whereby bilateral symmetry, which largely typifies the phyla, gave way to bilateral specialization. In short, specialization theory assumes that the type of neural organization underlying the unique mental functions of the left hemisphere is inappropriate for and even incompatible with the neural organization that sustains the cognitive style of the right hemisphere, and as a consequence, adaptive evolutionary forces provided that these distinct modes be distributed in separate hemispheres[33,41].

Intuitively, it is difficult to accept specialization theory. If the right half-brain processes information in a holistic, synthetic fashion, while the left processes information analytically, where and

how is it that these distinct and neurologically incompatible processing modes are integrated in the brain? Are we really to believe
that such basic processes as analysis and synthesis are not integral
facets of the cognitive repertoire of both cerebral hemispheres in
man?

Hardly, for specialization theory also fails when the processing requirements and the real, rather than the assumed, capacities
of the hemispheres are considered. While it is the right hemisphere
that is viewed as uniquely specialized for holistic, synthetic processing, the left hemisphere must surely utilize such processing
modes in extracting meaning from words, sentences, paragraphs,
and the like. On the other hand, while it is the left hemisphere that
is viewed as conceptual and logical, the right hemisphere has been
shown to be capable of logical and conceptual operations[42].

Specialization theory is also hard-pressed to explain the fact
that following extensive early damage to the left hemisphere, the
right is largely capable of sustaining linguistic development[43-47].
How is this the case if the right hemisphere has a genetically specified neurological scheme that is inappropriate for and incompatible
with the neural circuitry that sustains language?

Such considerations led us to review the split-brain studies
that provided the impetus for the view that the left hemisphere has
become specialized for analytic and verbal processing, while the
right has become specialized for holistic, Gestalt, synthetic, perceptual processing. We started with the idea that the right-
hemisphere advantage on the block-design task might represent a
superior capacity for response production, as suggested earlier[32],
rather than a visuospatial perceptual specialization, as is generally
assumed. We tested this notion by administering a lateralized visual–visual match test to P.S., using the block-design patterns.
The results of this simple experiment encouraged us to see if other
instances of a right-hemisphere advantage might also be sensitive
to slight methodological changes[48].

In the process of our studying this issue, it became apparent
that practically every demonstration of a right-hemisphere advantage in split-brain patients critically involved the hands as the
mode of either stimulus perception or response production. And,
as it turns out, our control experiments that deflated the right-

hemisphere advantage centered around minimizing the use of the hands.

In the following, we describe these control experiments, all of which were conducted on case P.S. Although these are but one-subject demonstrations, our general approach is first to show that P.S. performed like any other split-brain patient on several classic tasks when the test was administered in the traditional manner. We then show how the simple methodological change reversed the results of the experiment. Most important, however, is the interpretation of cerebral lateralization that emerged from these data.

MANIPULOSPATIAL ASPECTS OF CEREBRAL LATERALIZATION

One of the clearest and most dramatic demonstrations of hemisphere asymmetry results from the administration of the block-design task to split-brain patients[32]. On each trial, the patient is presented with four patterned cubes and a sample design (Figure 16) and is required to arrange the cubes manually to form the design. The performance of each hand is separately timed. The

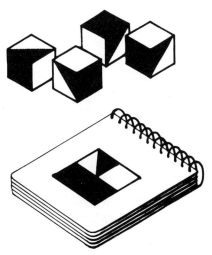

FIGURE 16. Block-design task. The subject arranges the four cubes to match the sample pattern. The performance of each hand is separately timed.

data resulting from the administration of this task to P.S. are shown in Table 1. The left hand consistently constructed the design faster than the preferred right hand, suggesting a clear right-hemisphere superiority, as previously reported for split-brain patients. The question remained, however, whether the left-hemisphere deficit lay primarily in the realm of stimulus perception or in the realm of response production. We approached this question first by tachistoscopically lateralizing the block-design patterns to one hemisphere or the other and having P.S. select the matching design after visually inspecting the three choices (Figure 17). On each of the 12 trials, the correct choice was selected regardless of the hemisphere tested. Several months later, we again lateralized block-design patterns, but this time we had P.S. construct the designs. Following left hemisphere exposure, the right hand constructed 1 of the 6 designs correctly, and after right hemisphere exposure, the left hand completed 5 of the 6 designs correctly. Taken together, these data suggest that both hemispheres are capable of appreciating the visuospatial aspects of the block-design task, but the right hemisphere is vastly if not absolutely superior to the left in constructing the perceived relations by manipulating the items appropriately.

Consider another dramatic instance of hemisphere asymme-

TABLE 1. Performance of Left and Right
Hands on Block-Design Task

| | Time (in Seconds) | |
Design	Left Hand	Right Hand
1.	11	18
2.	[a]	74[b]
3.	13	36
4.	12	69
5.	15	95[b]
6.	25	74[c]

[a] Design not completed within time limit (120 seconds).
[b] Subject gave up before end of time limit.
[c] Correct design was constructed but in wrong orientation.

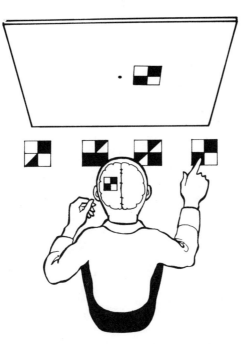

FIGURE 17. Lateralized block-design patterns. The sample patterns are tachisto-scopically lateralized to one hemisphere or the other, and the subject points to the matching stimulus.

try. P.S. could draw a cube with either hand prior to surgery. Fol-lowing commissurotomy, however, as shown in Figure 18, the drawing produced by the preferred right hand lacked the spatial completeness of the cube produced by the left hand, thus confirm-ing the classic hemisphere difference[30]. Again, it was not clear whether the right-hand deficit resulted because the left hemisphere did not know what a cube was or because it simply could not draw a cube.

When the word *cube* was flashed to his left hemisphere, P.S. readily selected a match-stick model of a Necker cube and ignored a model of the cube that had been drawn by his right hand. While this observation alone is not very significant, it is consistent with the recent finding that both hemispheres of split-brain patients have the capacity to appreciate the spatial relations of Euclidean geome-

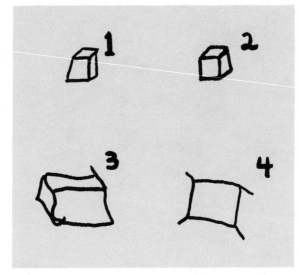

FIGURE 18. Cube drawing before and after commissurotomy. Preoperatively, P.S. could draw a cube with either hand. Postoperatively, however, the preferred right hand performed poorly. (1 = left hand pre-op; 2 = right hand pre-op; 3 = left hand post-op; 4 = right hand post-op.)

try[73]. Taken together, these observations suggest that the left hemisphere can indeed apprehend the simple spatial features of a cube but, as with the block-design task, has difficulty in appropriately representing spatiality using a manual or manipulative response.

Other classic split-brain experiments, which have not required a manipulative response as such, have also suggested that the capacity for spatial appreciation is special to the right hemisphere. However, the following observations suggest that even in these experiments, the right-hemisphere advantage is closely tied to manipulative activities.

For example, Milner and Taylor very convincingly demonstrated a right-hemisphere advantage in the perception and memory of complex tactual patterns (wire figures)[38] (Figure 19). They suggested that this advantage represents a superior capacity of the

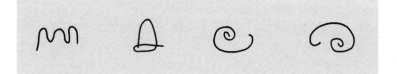

FIGURE 19. Wire-figures task. The subject manually explores one figure and subsequently is required to retrieve that figure, using the same hand, from the group of four figures. Each hand is tested separately. Figure adapted from Milner and Taylor[38].

right hemisphere for spatial processing, and thus should exist independent of the sensory modality tested.

We administered the wire-figures task to P.S. under different conditions. In the tactual–tactual condition, he was required to palpate a figure with one hand and then immediately select the same figure from a group of four, using the same hand. In this condition, the left hand correctly retrieved all four figures, but the right hand performed at chance. This finding confirms the results of Milner and Taylor. The other condition, which was not reported on by Milner and Taylor, was administered to test the generality of the right-hemisphere advantage. In the visual–visual condition, sketches of the figures were tachistoscopically lateralized, and P.S. was required to point to the correct figure following visual inspection of the choices. In this condition, both hemispheres performed perfectly. Thus, when the manipulative system was excluded from the wire-figures task, the classic left–right dichotomy found for the manipulative (tactual–tactual) condition disappeared.

Finally, consider an experiment by Nebes, who found that the right hemisphere of split-brain patients was vastly superior to the left on a task designed to measure the capacity of the separated hemispheres to process spatial information synthetically[36]. The patients were required to examine manually three geometric designs while looking at a sketch of one of the items in a fragmented form. The fragment was constructed by the cutting up and separating of one of the designs, with the original orientation and relative position of the parts maintained, however. The subject's task was to determine which one of the three items being tactually examined matched the fragmented stimulus. The right hand essentially performed at chance (33%), while the left-hand scores ranged between 75% and 90% correct.

We altered the design of this experiment so that the synthetic demands of the task would be emphasized, as opposed to the manipulative demands (see Figure 20). P.S. visually examined three fragmented forms on each trial. Subsequently, a whole design, which matched one of the fragments, was tachistoscopically lateralized to the left or the right hemisphere. Each hemisphere received 20 trials. Under these conditions, the left hemisphere correctly identified the fragment that the lateralized whole stimulus represented on 17 of 20 trials (85%), and the right hemisphere was correct on 20 of 20 trials. Thus, when the manipulative aspects of the figural unification task were circumvented, and the synthetic processing demands were emphasized, both hemispheres in P.S. proved capable of high-level performance.

These data suggest that the superior performance of the right

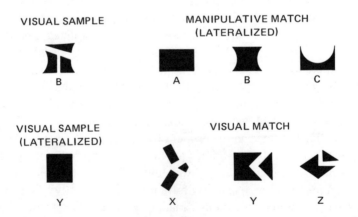

FIGURE 20. Fragmented-stimulus task. The top row shows the design of the experiment, as administered by Nebes[36]. The subject manually explores the three forms while looking at the fragmented visual sample. Here, the manipulative demands are stressed. The bottom row shows our nonmanipulative modification of the design. Following the lateralized visual presentation of a whole form, the subject visually examines three fragmented forms.

hemisphere of split-brain patients on a variety of tasks is related to the critical involvement of manual activities in the test design. This manipulospatial superiority includes the perception of spatial stimuli and the production of spatial responses.

The importance of these observations is highlighted by the fact that virutally every demonstration of a qualitative right-hemisphere advantage (which means here that the left hemisphere performs at or near chance, while the right performs at high levels) in split-brain patients has involved manipulospatial activities[34-36,38,73]. Since our data suggest that the hemispheres differ qualitatively along the manipulospatial dimension, a reasonable hypothesis is that manipulospatial involvement accounts for these qualitative differences. However, many of the studies have involved visual as well as manipulospatial functions, and our hypothesis does not rule out the possibility that the right hemisphere may have a relative (as opposed to a qualitative) edge over the left for complex visual perception. In fact, data to be reviewed later suggest that this is indeed the case. However, for the moment, we will put such relative differences aside and instead focus on the nature of the manipulospatial function. In doing so, we will uncover what we feel are some important clues to the origin of cerebral lateralization in man.

The Nature of Manipulospatial Activities

While we use the term *manipulospatial* to describe activities that would otherwise be called motor and perceptual functions, we feel that the idea of a manipulospatial mechanism transcends the simple notions of perceptual and motor functions. It is, after all, the preferred right hand that is deficient in manipulospatial skills in split-brain patients. In fact, we view the manipulospatial function as neither perceptual nor motor per se but rather as the mechanism by which a spatial context is mapped onto the perceptual and motor activities of the hands. On the efferent side, we are referring to the activities involved in drawing, arranging, constructing, or otherwise manipulating items so that the parts are in the appropriate relationship to one another. Concerning the afferent mechanisms, we are primarily referring to functions similar to what Gibson has described as "active touch"[75], which basically means the active, exploratory manipulations involved in the evaluation of the spatiotemporal features of complex haptic stimuli. Thus, we view manipulospatial mechanisms as a means of actively exploring and altering the spatial environment by using the hands.

We feel that the manipulospatial function is part of the more basic neural mechanism by which the organism maintains and actively utilizes the spatial relationship between its body and the surrounding spatial environment. While all animals must certainly possess this basic mechanism, the manipulative aspect is likely to have been associated with the evolution of the primates. Although there are several theories of primate origins, each emphasizes the importance of refinements in the functions of the extremities[49-54]. In particular, claws were replaced by tactually sensitive, grasping extremities, which expanded the primate's capacity for perceiving the world, moving skillfully among the slender branches of the arboreal environment, and manually capturing prey[51-53]. Thus, the hands essentially became specialized for prehension and took over the snout's functions of manipulation and food gathering. Also, changes in the visual apparatus allowing extensive binocular vision provided the early primates with a means of accurately localizing points in space and gauging distance in both manual prey-catching and arboreal locomotion[53]. Thus, it can be said that an increased capacity for interacting with the spatial environment typifies primate evolution. While the visual adaptation is similar to that seen in cats and owls[53], the manipulative specialization is largely a unique primate feature, with wide-ranging implication for subsequent evolutionary advances, as described later.

The Neural Substrate of Manipulospatiality

Physiological studies of nonhuman primates have recently shown that the awareness of the relationship of the animal's bodily parts to the spatial environment is a function of the inferior parietal lobule (IPL)[55,56]. In these experiments, it was found that many cells in IPL were activated by reaching and manipulatory movements. The neurons did not respond when the animal's arm was passively moved by the experimenter but only when the animal was actively reaching for or manipulating an object that was desired. In addition, the cells were generally contralateral and specific for particular points in the immediate surrounding space. Finally, these cells fired independently of the speed and latency of movement and thus were not simply motor neurons.

The conclusion from these studies is that the awareness of the body in relation to its spatial environment is represented in IPL, and this representation is used for the manual exploration of extrapersonal space. The identified properties of IPL neurons correlate well with manipulative adaptations associated with the phylogenetic emergence of the primates and furthermore suggest that in the monkey, the IPL of both hemispheres plays a critical role in the mediation of manipulospatial functions.

In man, damage to the right IPL has long been associated with manipulospatial deficits [2,5–7,11,57]. Although there have been reports suggesting manipulospatial deficits following left-hemisphere lesions, the deficits are generally less severe and seem to differ qualitatively from the right syndrome [5,7,10,13,14,57]. In addition, regardless of whether the lesion has been in the left or the right hemisphere, the preferred right hand has generally been tested.

Split-brain studies have shown how critical a factor hand use is and have suggested further that it is mainly the right hemisphere that houses the neural substrate of manipulospatiality. It is as if the left-hemisphere deficit goes beyond a simple lesion effect, and in-

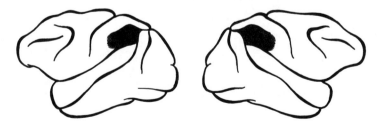

FIGURE 21. The inferior parietal lobule in the left and right hemisphere of the monkey brain (see text for explanation).

stead the lesion serves to callosally disconnect the right IPL from the manipulospatial representation in the posterior left hemisphere and thus from the motor regions of the left hemisphere that control the right hand. That the left-hemisphere syndrome is often described as a "milder" version of the right syndrome suggests the possibility that the right hemisphere is homolaterally directing the manipulospatial activities of the right hand. This is also indicated by P.S.'s performance on the block-design task, where the right hand, while clearly less efficient than the left, could construct several of the designs when the sample patterns were available in free vision, and thus were seen by both hemispheres, but when only the left hemisphere saw the design, the right-hand performance deteriorated substantially. Thus, it could be the inefficiency of homolateral control that gives the appearance of mild constructional apraxia in left-hemisphere damaged patients.

Why is it that the human left hemisphere seems to be minimally involved in manipulsopatial functions? After all, in nonhuman primates, the IPL of each hemisphere maintains a contralateral body–environment spatial map. In man, however, the left IPL is tied up, in a synaptic sense, with linguistic functions[58] (Figure 22). The lesion of the left hemisphere that produces the manipulospatial-like defect is, accordingly, not in the IPL but instead seems to involve the cell populations that surround the language-

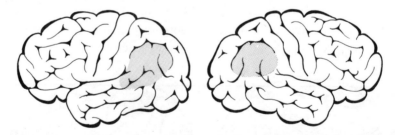

FIGURE 22. Language versus manipulospatiality in the human cerebrum. In the right half-brain, the presumed neural substrate of manipulospatiality (the inferior parietal lobule) is shaded. The shaded area in the left hemisphere represents the language-comprehension regions of the parietotemporal junction (see text for explanation).

comprehension regions of the IPL and the remainder of the parietotemporal junction[57].

These cytoarchitectonic considerations, in conjunction with
our clinical observations, graphically suggest that the phylogenetic
emergence of human language resulted in a redistribution of function in the posterior association region of the left hemisphere. That
is, synaptic space previously (in a phyletic sense) devoted to manipulospatial functions in the left hemisphere was sacrificed in the
process of acquiring language. Manipulospatial functions, however, managed to retain a minimal representation in the surrounding association cortex. We thus hypothesize that it is by way of
this representation and its callosal connections that the right IPL
essentially sustains the entirety of manipulospatial appreciation in
man.

These observations concerning the probable neural substrate
of manipulospatial functions have important implications for the
way we view lateralized processes in the human brain. We feel
that the right-hemisphere advantage on manipulospatial tasks may
not be attributable to an evolutionarily superior right hemisphere
but instead to a disadvantaged left hemisphere. That is, the superior performance of the right hemisphere on these tasks may not
reflect the overall, specialized cognitive style of the right hemisphere but instead may represent definable, localized processing
inefficiencies in the posterior left hemisphere due to the intruding
presence of language in the parietotemporal junction.

The Language–Manipulospatial Relationship

Why should language and manipulospatiality compete for the
same synaptic space? One interesting hypothesis is based on the
theory that language emerged out of tool using[59]. As the theory
goes, tool using precipitated a focus on objects, and object naming
was the end result. Yet, it would seem that the more basic factor
involved was the emergence of a means of manipulating objects
that were to become tools. Nevertheless, tool using in defense,
play, construction, and foodgathering is certainly a manipulospa-

tial derivative and depends on various combinations of tactual, visual, and spatial integration. Similar cross-modal interactions have been postulated as the basis of language[58], which is thought by some to have emerged as object naming[58-60].

So, it is clear that manipulospatiality and language are complexly related. Manipulospatial abilities may have provided the basis for primitive language (object naming), and both language and manipulospatiality require similar neural mechanisms (cross-modal convergence). These observations suggest why language and manipulospatiality might demand the same neural substrate.

Competition for Synaptic Space

Since manipulospatiality is the phylogenetic resident of the inferior parietal lobule, the burden is on language to acquire space. One way this could happen would be for language to be programmed to emerge in development prior to manipulospatiality. As it turns out, language does emerge early. By the second postnatal year, language is a viable force for parents to enjoy and contend with. In contrast, manipulospatial functions come in much later. As Inhelder and Piaget have shown, the ability to draw and copy geometric designs and manually appreciate spatial forms is a late-developing skill (sixth or seventh year)[61]. This later development correlates well with the timetable by which language, which starts out bilaterally in development, becomes largely left-lateralized in most right-handers[62,63]. Thus, manipulospatiality may be held in check until language is firmly committed to the left hemisphere, or manipulospatiality may simply be a late-developing function. In any event, by the time manipulospatiality does emerge, language has tied up (in a synaptic sense) the left parieto-temporal junction, which places the burden of maintaining the body–space map entirely on the right IPL.

While the foregoing suggestions presume some fancy synaptic footwork during ontogeny, recent experiments concerning synaptic reorganization suggest the possible mechanisms involved. Schneider has shown that a developing projection system can be directed to a cell population with which it does not normally interact and that the anomalous projection can actively compete with the normal projection for terminal space[64]. By inference, it would seem that if the anomalous projection arrived first and tied up the terminal space the later-arriving normal projection would be prevented from forming synapses.

Presumably, nature is as clever an experimenter as man. By simply arranging neural maturation so that language synapses are formed prior to manipulospatial synapses, language could effectively tie up the left parietotemporal junction. As a consequence, manipulospatiality would essentially be excluded from forming synapses in this region, and in addition, less space would be available for other nonlanguage functions of the left posterior neocortex (i.e., visual and auditory perception). This simple hypothesis suggests an explanation for why the right hemisphere has a relative

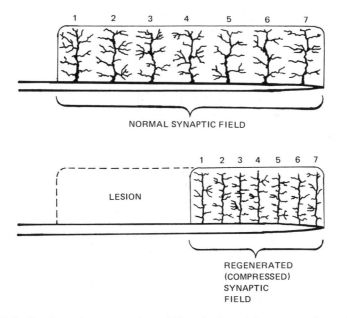

FIGURE 23. Synaptic compression. Although the total amount of terminal space is reduced, the system terminates fully in the compressed space. Figure adapted from Schneider[64].

advantage on some visual and auditory perceptual tasks (we will return to perceptual lateralization in a later section).

Before we leave this topic, it is important to point out other relevant findings from Schneider's developmental research[64]. If one eye and the ipsilateral tectum of a hamster are lesioned during early development, the optic tract from the undamaged eye, having been evicted from the damaged tectum, recrosses the cerebral midline to synapse on the vacated, undamaged tectum. Moreover, if part of one tectum is removed at an early age, the retinal fibers reorganize and project fully upon the undamaged part, which results in a compression of the retinotopic map (see Figure 23). These data show how during an early critical period a lateralized neural system (the optic tract projection to the tectum) can be redirected to the side of the brain that it does not normally interact with. Moreover, these data show how early damage to a neural system can serve as a stimulus that makes it possible for the brain to carry out normal functions in less than the normal amount of space. Taken together, such observations suggest an explanation for the fact that after early removal of the left hemisphere in humans, the right hemisphere can acquire language in addition to its normal repertoire of nonlanguage functions. The early lesion requires that all cortical functions be organized in one hemisphere, and compression of synaptic space makes this possible.

Thus, we suggest two developmental models of competition for synaptic space between language and manipulospatial functions. In normal development, language competes by emerging early and tying up space before manipulospatiality sets in. However, when the system is pathologically perturbed, leaving one half-brain to carry out all functions, synaptic compression allows more to be done in less space. While these models are clearly speculative, they certainly suggest an intriguing and empirically viable interpretation of the facts of cerebral lateralization.

Origins

Throughout the preceding discussion, two assumptions have been explicit. One is that language is lateralized and the other is that it is left-lateralized. While counter examples for both of these assumptions are readily available, they are just as readily interpreted by the theory.

The important point from our point of view is that the key factor determining functional asymmetry is where language settles both between and within the cerebral hemispheres. As a consequence of where language is, the prototypical primate brain plan is altered. To the extent that language uses up space within a hemisphere, nonlanguage functions of that half-brain must sacrifice space. Thus, most if not all measurable instances of lateralized processing, according to the theory, are really by-products of the lateralization of linguistic mechanisms, and in the next chapter, we will consider why language is lateralized. For the present, we would like simply to reemphasize that the dramatic dichotomy of lateralization seems to be language versus manipulospatiality. In this regard, it is interesting to note that one of the first reports documenting specific cognitive deficits following right-hemisphere damage pointed out the manipulative nature of the spatial defect[2]. This early finding, which we seem to have rediscovered, has been largely overshadowed by an emphasis on the role of the right hemisphere in perceptual processing, the topic to which we now turn.

PERCEPTUAL PROCESSING AND CEREBRAL LATERALIZATION

A variety of normal and clinical studies of visual and auditory processing have suggested that the nonverbal perceptual skills of the right half-brain exceed those of the left. As these studies were largely stimulated by the split-brain data on lateralized mechanisms, the findings came to be interpreted within and viewed as supporting the hemisphere-specialization theoretical framework.

In light of our observations and speculations concerning the manipulospatial aspects of lateralization, it seems useful to reconsider the data viewed as supporting the idea that the right hemisphere in man is specialized for perceptual processing. Our goal in this section is thus to evaluate critically the nature of hemisphere differences in perceptual capacities for the purpose of determining whether such differences warrant the view that the neurological circuitry of the left hemisphere is inappropriate for and incompatible with the mechanisms of perceptual processing. We will focus on the visual modality and will consider the results of studies of split-brain, brain-damaged, and normal subjects.

Split-Brain Studies

Most of the split-brain studies that have assessed the visual perceptual capacities of the separated hemispheres have been confounded by the involvement of manipulospatial activities in the test design[32-36,38,73]. Our data suggest that the involvement of the hands in these tests accounts for much of the asymmetry observed. This is not to say that the hemispheres are equal in their visual perceptual capacities. As we observed on the fragmented-figures task, circumvention of the manipulative mode did not completely dissolve the right-hemisphere advantage. What it did seem to do, however, was convert a qualitative hemisphere difference into a relative advantage.

There have been some, though not many, studies of visual processing in split-brain patients that have not been confounded by manipulospatial involvement. For example, in one study, the separated hemispheres were required to judge whether arrays of dots seemed to form vertical or horizontal lines[37]. The right hemisphere was found to be superior to the left, and these results were attributed to the specialization of the right half-brain for Gestalt perception. However, both hemispheres were substantially above chance. In addition, it is worth noting that the right-hemisphere advantage was obtained by the use of a 20-msec visual exposure, which is considerably lower than the 100-msec to 150-msec exposure typically used in split-brain experiments. Was such a short exposure necessary to achieve this effect? If so, the hemisphere differences in this study, which were not very impressive to begin with, are of questionable importance. Finally, other factors besides a perceptual superiority of the right could have contributed to the hemisphere differences. For example, virtually all left-hemisphere errors were of the "false-positive" type, which, within the framework of signal-detection theory[76], suggests the possibility that the left-hemisphere error rate was inflated, not because of inferior perceptual capacities but because of "response bias." This idea is strengthened by the fact that in a study of visual recognition, Kimura[23] observed that the errors of the right-damaged group (which means the group with the intact left hemisphere) was also accounted for by false positives.

More dramatic is the observation of right-hemisphere dominance on the bilateral chimeric stimulus task. Levy, Trevarthen, and Sperry[39] presented split-brain patients with two half-stimuli joined at the midline of visual fixation on each trial. Regardless of whether the stimuli were nameable (such as common objects) or resistant to verbal identification (such as complex visual patterns or faces), the choice item corresponding to the half-stimulus seen by the right hemisphere was nearly always selected, as long as a simple pointing response was required. While this effect has been interpreted as indicative of the superior perceptual capacities of the right hemisphere, it must be emphasized that right dominance simply involved control over the response mechanism, for it was shown that although the left hemisphere failed to respond, it nevertheless perceived its stimulus. As such, the dramatic effect of right dominance is of minimal importance to questions concerning the perceptual capacities of the hemispheres. Furthermore, recent observations on case P.S. suggest that right dominance may be a by-product of the postoperative recovery involved in learning to live with a split brain[77] (Figure 24).

Of more relevance to the present discussion is the claim of Levy *et al.* that although both hemispheres formed visual percepts, each hemisphere used a unique perceptual strategy. The left supposedly used an analytic, verbal strategy, while the right employed a holistic strategy. This conclusion, which was based on the verbal reports of the subjects as well as on an analysis of the errors obtained by the hemispheres on different tests, is not without problems.

In the first place, if you ask the patient—which is to say, the

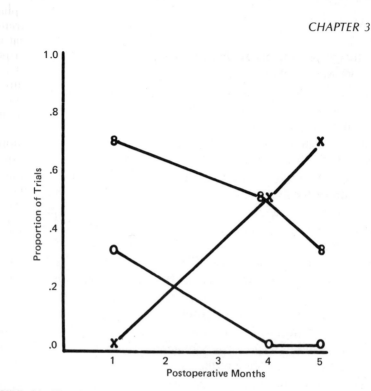

FIGURE 24. The development of right dominance on the bilateral chimeric stimulus task. When chimeric tests were administered to P.S. during the first postoperative month, performance was dominated by bilateral responses (**8—8**). Each hemisphere selected the appropriate matching stimulus on a majority of the trials. While the left hemisphere (O—O) dominated performance on some trials, the right (**X—X**) never did. In the fourth postoperative month, right dominance occurred as often as bilateral responding. By the fifth month, right dominance seemed to be the preferred mode. These observations on case P.S. suggest the possibility that right dominance on the chimeric test is not characteristic of the way the normal brain processes information, as right dominance does not develop until late in the postoperative recovery period. Perhaps right dominance reflects a strategy employed by the brain to cope with interhemispheric rivalry instituted by the split condition.

left hemisphere—to describe what he saw, his verbal description of a complex visual stimulus will necessarily be analytic and piecemeal, even if the left hemisphere has fully perceived the item as a "whole." A verbal response from the left hemisphere cannot be viewed as a true index of the perceptual status of that half-brain. Second, the error-score analysis of the chimeric data was based on the verbal performance of the left hemisphere and the pointing performance of the right. The right simply had to select one of the choices available by pointing. In contrast, the left had to learn the names that went with faces or other complex visual patterns and then had to recall the name from memory after seeing the stimulus. The difficulty of the left hemisphere's task relative to the right's could clearly account, at least in part, for the inferior performance of the left hemisphere on the "nonverbal" tests. As an added control, however, Levy *et al.* administered one of the complex pattern tests as a single-field, whole-stimulus test, on which both hemispheres responded by pointing to the correct choice. While the right hemisphere had a clear, though relative, advantage, it is suspicious that only one of the four patients involved in the other phases of the study was reported on.

All things considered, the split-brain studies are of little help in specifying the nature and extent of hemisphere differences in perceptual mechanisms. While there is certainly no conclusive evidence for qualitative differences in visual capacities, there is the suggestion of a right-hemisphere relative superiority, but methodological considerations complicate the data interpretation.

Normal Studies

Using the EEG technique to measure hemisphere differences in normals, Galin and Ornstein found significant left–right differences in alpha blocking on verbal and visual tasks[70]. Not surprisingly, the right hemisphere seemed to show less activity than the left on verbal tasks. On the visual task, the reverse was found. However, the visual task was the block-design task, which we view as a manipulospatial task, and as we have seen, there are good reasons why the hemisphere differences should have occurred[48]. It is also not surprising that when Ornstein expanded his tests to include purely visual tasks, he failed to find left–right differences[71]. Similarly, Donchin, using the evoked potentials technique, has been unable to substantiate claims of perceptual asymmetry[82].

A variety of studies of normal subjects using recognition[25,26] and reaction-time[69,72,79] procedures have found visual-field effects that are suggestive of a right-hemisphere superiority in perceiving visual stimuli that are resistant to verbal encoding. It should be pointed out, however, that every worker in the field knows of more perceptual tests that do not yield the effect than do. In addition, while positive findings are likely to be published, failures to find evidence suggesting hemispheric differences, given the current mind-set in neuropsychology, are viewed as a design problem rather than as a reflection of the reality of neural function. Finally, the differences, when found, are generally small and statistical, and while they suggest a relative advantage on some dimension, they certainly fail to support in any convincing way the view that the hemispheres differ qualitatively in visual capacities. Similar criticisms are relevant to studies of hemispheric differences in auditory and musical perception[19,22,80].

Clinical Studies of Visual Recognition

Observations on visual recognition following lateralized brain damage show greater deficits following right-hemisphere damage, thus suggesting that the right half-brain plays a greater role than the left in visual processing[15,17,20,23,24,66,68]. These studies also suggest, however, that the right-hemisphere advantage mainly surfaces when the tasks tax the discriminative and integrative capacities of the hemispheres[23,66,68]. The interpretation here would seem to be that both the left and right half-brains have substantial capacities for visual recognition, with the right excelling mainly when the upper perceptual limits are tested.

So when the results of normal, split-brain, and other clinical studies are critically examined, we find that there is little support for the view that the neural organization of the left hemisphere is incompatible with the mechanisms of perceptual processing. In other words, although the right hemisphere shows a relative advantage on some perceptual tests, perceptual processing is clearly the business of both half-brains. How else could the left hemisphere of split-brain patients function in the world?

The implications of these varied observations for left–right brain organization are simple and straightforward. In our earlier discussion of manipulospatial functions, we suggested that as a result of the development of linguistic mechanisms, the left hemisphere sacrifices space and efficiency in mediating manipulospatial functions. But language comprehension occupies the entire left parietotemporal junction, not just the inferior parietal lobule. Immediately surrounding this junction in the left hemisphere are the association areas of the visual, auditory, and somatosensory systems. It is our view that these systems also suffer, though mainly at the upper perceptual limits, from the intruding presence of language. Consequently, we feel that the qualitatively superior manipulospatial and the relatively superior perceptual skills of the right hemisphere arise as a by-product of the fact that language is usually in the left and thus do not represent evolved specializations of the right.

LOOSE ENDS

The experienced student of brain asymmetry is at this point no doubt wondering how our model accounts for certain clinical syndromes, thus far ignored, that result from lateralized cerebral damage. Before considering specific points, it is important to note that it has long been recognized that the symptoms produced by brain pathology do not necessarily coincide with the functions of the damaged tissue. With this warning in mind, let's examine a couple of these syndromes.

Unilateral spatial agnosia involves the inattention to or the neglect of one half of visual space. In the vast majority of cases reported, the disorder occurs as a consequence of lesions in the parietooccipital region of the right hemisphere, and it is the left half of space that is ignored[4,5,9,74]. Patients manifesting neglect will often bump into objects that are unattended to on the left side of their paths. They will frequently be unable to find their way around the corridors of the hospital, always making right turns, acting as though left turns do not exist. When performing simple constructive tasks such as drawing patterns or arranging items in a systematic way, they frequently ignore the left side of the pattern, completing only the right side. When reading, they will start in the middle of a line, again ignoring the left side. If asked to point to the middle of a horizontal line, they will invariably point somewhere in the middle of the right side, which is probably very close to the middle of the line that is actually perceived.

Thus, neglect actually accounts for the poor performance of right-damaged patients on a variety of "spatial" tasks. In many cases, it is not that the patient has really lost the capacity to perceive spatial relations, but instead that the patient neglects part of space and thus performs poorly on tasks requiring the use of the neglected space, while still manifesting intact visuospatial skills in the unneglected space.

While a variety of theories have surfaced to explain neglect, most agree that neglect represents a disturbance in the mechanism by which one half of space is attended to. This suggests that attention to one side of space requires such a mechanism. If this is so, we are then faced with the problem of explaining how the right side of space is normally attended to, as neglect usually involves the left side of space.

Since the left hemisphere of split-brain patients can and does attend to the right side of space, we have no alternative but to accept the conclusion that each hemisphere has its own mechanisms for attending to the contralateral half of space. It would appear that the parietooccipital region plays an important role in these mechanisms, and our guess is that it does so by mediating between the cortical sensory and association areas and various subcortical structures, including the tectum, which has for some time been implicated in multimodal attentional processes.

Given this model, we propose two possible explanations for the rarity of unilateral inattention following left-hemisphere lesions. Perhaps neglect of the right side of space is seldom seen because damage to the left-parietooccipitotemporal junction produces such severe distortions of consciousness (because of extensive linguistic losses) that it becomes difficult, if not impossible, to assess more subtle disturbances like neglect. Alternatively, the invasion of the left-parietooccipitotemporal region by linguistic functions may force the attentional circuitry to occupy more posterior cortical areas. The lesion leading to neglect of the right half of space would thus be in or close to the left-occipital cortex. As occipital lesions are far more likely than more anterior lesions to render the patient blind in the opposite half-field, and the difficulty in assessing neglect escalates with the degree of visual field defect, left-lesioned patients would be less likely to show the syndrome.

Next consider the syndrome called prosopagnosia, or face agnosia. Prosopagnosic patients, as the theory goes, selectively lose the capacity to recognize faces following parietooccipital damage in the right hemisphere. As a consequence, the view has emerged that the right hemisphere is the face perceiver. While this conclusion may be based on a real clinical phenomenon, it is inconsistent with a variety of other lines of evidence. In the first place, although the clinical disorder involves the inability to recognize familiar faces, experimental evidence from normal subjects has shown a left-hemisphere advantage on a familiar face recognition test[81]. Second, split-brain patients are able to associate familiar faces with names, which must be done in their left hemisphere. Third, when unfamiliar faces are used in perceptual tests, unselected brain-damaged patients show more of a deficit following right hemisphere damage[24]. These latter results, however, mirror the results seen on other visual perceptual tests—a relative right-hemisphere advantage. Consequently, the evidence fails to justify the conclusion that face perception is a unique capacity of the right hemisphere. As with so many other syndromes resulting from focal damage, it is difficult to use the behavioral defect as valid index of functional localization, particularly when the syndrome is as rare and little understood as prosopagnosia.

CONCLUSIONS

The theory of hemisphere specialization has attracted much attention in recent years. A large part of its popular appeal would seem to involve its affirmation of man's uniqueness in the animal kingdom. While we do not question the uniqueness of man, we do take issue with the view that through evolutionary wisdom each hemisphere in man has been separately endowed with a neural organization that is incompatible with the type of processing that occurs in the other half-brain. We prefer the view that what has become uniquely specialized and genetically specified in the course of human neural evolution is a potential for the expression of linguistic functions. The actual expression of these functions appears to be experientally dependent, with the final location being secondarily determined and subject to ontogenetic as well as genetic factors. Moreover, we feel that where linguistic functions finally settle down in the brain during development alters the prototypical primate brain plan so that homologous areas in opposite hemispheres come to carry out different functions. Thus, according to this view, lateralized functions do not reflect the genetically specified cognitive styles of the hemispheres but instead represent specific, localized differences in cerebral organization that are closely tied to the inter- and intrahemispheric localization of linguistic mechanisms. Viewed in this manner, the cerebral hemispheres in man do not oppose each other but instead work together to maintain the integrity of mental functioning.

REFERENCES

1. J. H. Jackson, 1958, *Selected Writings of John Hughlings Jackson,* J. Taylor (Ed.), New York, Basic Books.
2. T. Weisenburg and K. E. McBride, 1935, *Aphasia: A Clinical and Psychological Study,* New York, Commonwealth Fund.
3. J. M. Neilsen, Unilateral cerebral dominance as related to mind blindness, *Arch. Neurol. Psychiatr. 38:*108–135.
4. R. Brain, 1941, Visual disorientation with special reference to the lesions of the right cerebral hemisphere, *Brain 64:*244–272.
5. A. Paterson and O. Zangwill, 1944, Disorders of visual space perception associated with lesions of the right cerebral hemisphere, *Brain 67:*331–358.
6. H. Hecaen, J. DeAjuriaguerra, and J. Massonnet, 1951, Les troubles visuoconstructifs par lésion pariétooccipitale droite; Role des perturbations vestibulaires, *Encéphale 6:*533–562.
7. M. Critchley, 1953, *The Parietal Lobes,* London, Edward Arnold.

8. J. Semmes, S. Weinstein, L. Ghent, and H. L. Teuber, 1955, Spatial orientation in man after cerebral injury: Analyses by locus of lesion, *J. Psychol.* *39:*227–244.

9. N. S. Battersby, M. B. Bender, M. Pollack, and R. L. Kahn, 1956, Unilateral "spatial agnosia" (inattention), *Brain 79:*68–93.

10. J. McFie and O. L. Zangwill, 1960, Visual-constructive disabilities associated with lesions of the left hemisphere, *Brain 83:*243–260.

11. M. Piercy and V. O. G. Smyth, 1962, Right hemisphere dominance for certain non-verbal intellectual skills, *Brain 85:*775–790.

12. H. L. Teuber, 1963, Space perception and its disturbance after brain injury in man, *Neuropsychologia 1:*47–57.

13. G. Arrigoni and E. De Renzi, 1964, Constructional apraxia and hemispheric locus of lesion, *Cortex (Milano) 1:*170–197.

14. E. K. Warrington, M. James, and M. Kinsbourne, 1966, Drawing disability in relation to laterality of cerebral lesion, *Brain 89:*53–82.

15. E. De Renzi, P. Faglioni, and H. Spinnler, 1968, The performance of patients with unilateral brain damage on face recognition tasks, *Cortex 4:*17–34.

16. E. De Renzi, P. Faglioni, and G. Scotti, 1970, Hemispheric contribution to exploration of space through the visual and tactile modality, *Cortex 6:*191–203.

17. E. De Renzi, P. Faglioni, and G. Scotti, 1971, Judgment of spatial orientation in patients with focal brain damage, *J. Neurol. Neurosurg. Psychiatry 34:*489.

18. B. Milner, 1958, Psychological deficits produced by temporal lobe excision, *Res. Publ. Assoc. Res. Nerv. Ment. Dis. 36:*244–257.

19. B. Milner, 1962, Laterality effects in audition, in: V. B. Mountcastle (Ed.), *Interhemispheric Relations and Cerebral Dominance,* Baltimore, Johns Hopkins Press.

20. B. Milner, 1968, Visual recognition and recall after right temporal lobe excision in man, *Neuropsychologia 6:*191–209.

21. B. Milner, 1972, Interhemispheric differences in the localization of psychological processes in man, *Br. Med. Bull. 27:*272–277.

22. D. Kimura, 1961, Cerebral dominance and the perception of verbal stimuli, *Can. J. Psychol. 15:*166–171.

23. D. Kimura, 1963, Right temporal lobe damage: Perception of unfamiliar stimuli after damage, *Arch. Neurol. 8:*264–271.

24. E. De Renzi and H. Spinnler, 1966, Facial recognition in brain-damaged patients: An experimental approach, *Neurol. 6:*145–153.

25. D. Kimura, 1966, Dual functional asymmetry of the brain in visual perception, *Neuropsychologia 4:*275–285.

26. D. Kimura and M. Durnford, 1974, Normal studies on the function of the right hemisphere in vision, in: S. J. Dimond and J. G. Beaumont (Eds.), *Hemisphere Function in the Human Brain,* New York, Halsted Press.

27. J. E. Bogen and P. J. Vogel, 1962, Cerebral commissurotomy: A case report, *Bull. Los Angeles Neurol. Soc. 27:*169.
28. M. S. Gazzaniga, J. E. Bogen, and R. W. Sperry, 1962, Some functional effects of sectioning the cerebral commissures in man, *Proc. Nat. Acad. Sci. 48:*1765–1769.
29. M. S. Gazzaniga, J. E. Bogen, and R. W. Sperry, 1963, Laterality effects in somesthesis following cerebral commissurotomy in man, *Neuropsychologia 1:*209–215.
30. M. S. Gazzaniga, J. E. Bogen, and R. W. Sperry, 1965, Observations on visual perception after disconnexion of the cerebral hemispheres in man, *Brain 88:*221.
31. M. S. Gazzaniga, J. E. Bogen, and R. W. Sperry, 1967, Dyspraxia following division of the cerebral commissures, *Arch. Neurol. 16:*606–612.
32. J. E. Bogen and M. S. Gazzaniga, 1965, Cerebral commissurotomy in man: Minor hemisphere dominance for certain visuo-spatial functions, *J. Neurosurg. 23:*394–399.
33. J. Levy-Agresti and R. W. Sperry, 1968, Differential perceptual capacities in major and minor hemispheres, *Proc. Nat. Acad. Sci. 61:*1151.
34. E. Zaidel and R. W. Sperry, 1973, Performance on Raven's colored progressive matrices tests by commissurotomy patients, *Cortex 9:*34.
35. R. Nebes, 1971, Superiority of the minor hemisphere in commissurotomized man for the perception of part–whole relations, *Cortex 7:*333–349.
36. R. Nebes, 1972, Dominance of the minor hemisphere in commissurotomized man on a test of figural unification, *Brain 95:*633–638.
37. R. Nebes, 1973, Perception of spatial relationships by the right and left hemispheres of commissurotomized man, *Neuropsychologia 11:*285–289.
38. B. Milner and L. Taylor, 1972, Right hemisphere superiority in tactile pattern-recognition after cerebral commissurotomy: Evidence for nonverbal memory, *Neuropsychologia 10:*1–15.
39. J. Levy, C. Trevarthen, and R. W. Sperry, 1972, Perception of bilateral chimeric figures following hemispheric deconnection, *Brain 95:*61–78.
40. J. E. Bogen, 1969, The other side of the brain, II: An appositional mind, *Bull. L.A. Neurol. Soc. 34:*135–162.
41. J. Levy, 1974, Psychobiological implications of bilateral asymmetry, in: S. J. Dimond and J. G. Beaumont (Eds.), *Hemisphere Function in the Human Brain,* New York, Halsted Press.
42. A. S. Glass, M. S. Gazzaniga, and D. Premack, 1973, Artificial language training in global aphasics, *Neuropsychologia 11:*95–103.
43. L. S. Basser, 1962, Hemiplegia of early onset and the faculty of speech with special reference to the effects of hemispherectomy, *Brain 85:*28–52.
44. J. W. Brown and H. Hecaen, 1976, Lateralization and language representation, *Neurology 26:*183–189.
45. A. Smith, 1969, Nondominant hemispherectomy, *Neurology 19:*422–445.

46. A. Smith and C. W. Burklund, 1966, Dominant hemispherectomy, *Science* *153:*1280.

47. M. Dennis and H. Whitaker, 1976, Language acquisition following hemide-cortication, *Brain Lang. 3:*404–433.

48. J. E. LeDoux, D. H. Wilson, and M. S. Gazzaniga, 1977, Manipulo-spatial aspects of cerebral lateralization: Clues to the origin of lateralization, *Neuropsychologia,* in press.

49. G. E. Smith, 1912, The evolution of man, *Smithson. Inst. Annu. Rep.* 553.

50. F. W. Jones, 1916, *Arboreal Man,* London, Edward Arnold.

51. W. D. Matthew, 1904, The arboreal ancestry of the mammalia, *Am. Nat. 38:*811.

52. W. E. Le Gros Clarke, 1970, *History of the Primates,* London, British Museum (Nat. His.).

53. M. Cartmill, 1974, Rethinking primate origins, *Science 184:*436–443.

54. T. Collins, 1921, *Trans. Ophthalmol. Soc. U. R. 41:*10.

55. J. Hyvarinen and A. Poranen, 1974, Function of the parietal associative area 7 as revealed from cellular discharges in alert monkeys, *Brain 97:*673–692.

56. V. B. Mountcastle, J. C. Lynch, A. Georgopoulos, H. Sakata, and C. Acuna, 1975, Posterior parietal association cortex of the monkey: command functions for operations within extrapersonal space, *J. Neurophysiol. 38:*871–871–909.

57. M. Piercy, H. Hecaen, and J. De Ajuriaguerra, 1960, Constructional apraxia associated with lesions of the right cerebral hemisphere, *Brain 67:*331–358.

58. N. Geschwind, 1965, Disconnexion syndromes in animals and man, *Brain 88:*237–294, 585–644.

59. S. L. Washburn and R. S. Harding, 1972, Evolution of primate behavior, in: P. Dolhinow (Ed.), *Primate Patterns,* New York, Holt, Rinehart, Winston.

60. D. Premack, 1975, On the origins of language, in: M. S. Gazzaniga and C. Blakemore (Eds.), *Handbook of Psychobiology,* New York, Academic Press.

61. B. Inhelder and J. Piaget, 1956, *Child's Conception of Space,* New York, Norton.

62. J. W. Brown and H. Hecaen, 1976, Lateralization and language represen-tation, *Neurology 26:*183–189.

63. O. L. Zangwill, 1975, Ontogeny of cerebral dominance in man, in: E. H. Lenneberg and E. Lenneberg (Eds.), *Foundations of Language Development,* New York, Academic Press.

64. G. E. Schneider, 1976, Growth of abnormal neural connections following focal brain lesions: Constraining factors and functional effects, in: W. H. Sweet, S. Obrader, and J. G. Martin Rodriguez (Eds.), *Neurosurgical Treatment in Psychiatry,* Baltimore, University Park Press.

65. E. De Renzi, P. Faglioni, and H. Spinnler, 1968, The performance of patients with unilateral brain damage on face recognition tasks, *Cortex 4:*17–34.

66. E. K. Warrington and M. James, 1967, Disorders of visual perception in patients with localized cerebral lesions. *Neuropsychologia (Oxford)* 5:253–266.
67. E. De Renzi and H. Spinnler, 1966, Facial recognition in brain-damaged patients: An experimental approach, *Neurology* 6:145–153.
68. E. De Renzi and H. Spinnler, 1966, Visual recognition in patients with unilateral cerebral disease, *J. Nerv. Ment. Dis. 142:*515–525.
69. G. Berlucchi, 1973, Cerebral dominance and interhemispheric communication in normal man, in: F. O. Schmitt (Ed.), *The Neurosciences: Third Study Program,* Cambridge, Mass.: MIT Press.
70. D. Galin and R. Ornstein, 1972, Lateral specialization of cognitive modes: An EEG study, *Psychophysiology* 9:412–418.
71. R. Ornstein, 1976, Lateral specialization in normals: Paper read at the Conference on evolution of lateralization of the brain, N.Y. Academy of Science, November, 1976.
72. G. Geffen, J. L. Bradshaw, and G. Wallace, 1971, Interhemispheric effects on reaction time to verbal and nonverbal stimuli, *J. Exp. Psychol.* 87:415–422.
73. L. Franco and R. W. Sperry, 1977, Hemisphere lateralization for cognitive processing of geometry, *Neuropsychologia 15:*107–113.
74. H. Hecaen, 1969, Aphasic, apraxic, and agnosic syndromes in right and left hemisphere lesions, in: P. J. Vinken and G. W. Bruyn (Eds.), *Handbook of Clinical Neurology,* Vol. 4, New York, Wiley.
75. J. J. Gibson, 1962, Observations on active touch, *Psychol. Rev. 69:*477–491.
76. D. M. Green and J. A. Swets, 1966, *Signal Detection Theory and Psychophysics,* New York, Wiley.
77. J. E. LeDoux and M. S. Gazzaniga, unpublished observation.
78. M. M. Gross, 1972, Hemisphere specialization for processing of visually presented verbal and spatial stimuli, *Percept. Psychophys. 12:*357–363.
79. G. Geffen, J. L. Bradshaw, and N. C. Nettleton, 1972, Hemisphere asymmetry: Verbal and spatial encoding of visual stimuli, *J. Exp. Psychol.* 95:25–31.
80. D. Kimura, 1964, Left–right differences in the perception of melodies, *Q. J. Exp. Psychol. 16:*355–356.
81. G. Berlucchi, 1974, Some features of interhemispheric communication of visual information in brain damaged cats and normal humans, in: F. Michel and B. Schott (Eds.), *Les syndrômes de disconnexion calleuse chez l'homme,* Lyon, France, Colloque International de Lyon.
82. E. Donchin, Personal communication.

Brain and Language

While it is happily the case that one of the main objectives of neuroscience is to understand how the brain manages such complex behaviors as language and speech, it is sadly apparent that the field is nowhere near setting limiting conditions for a theory of language as a result of possessing specific knowledge about neural networks. The literature to date mostly reflects correlations in the grossest terms. Lateralized damage or disconnections yield patients with a general loss of this or that kind, and in the main, these observations have not produced enough information for a theory of brain and language. Indeed, the *a priori* issue of whether a system that is handling such a complex phenomenon can be studied after it is placed in such total disarray, as is the case following brain damage, is largely ignored.

From a purely neurophysiological and neuroanatomical point of view, there is at present no knowledge of what it is that makes the nervous system capable of language and speech. With respect to language, which here means the capacity to assign symbols to objects, events, concepts, and the like and to represent them in a way that carries the agent's intent to another organism, the essential biological capacity is particularly mystifying. As we shall see, this deep-core cognitive capacity seems resistant to massive brain damage in man and indeed is newly discovered to be present in chimpanzees and perhaps even lower animals. As a result, the old tactic of analyzing the gross anatomical discontinuities between man's brain as compared to the brain of the chimp and other animals no longer seems to be a fruitful enterprise, since the essential difference between these two groups on the language dimension is no longer clear. The uniqueness of man appears to be in the areas of speech production and reception.

In clinical studies, there have been a variety of phenomena noted following brain damage. Here, a series of well-known and striking abnormalities appear with a high degree of regularity as a consequence of discrete lesions. The problem has been, however, what to do with them. It is not unlike the problem of a radio engineer listening to the squeaks and squawks of a broken radio. No matter how reliable and accurate his measures might be of the radio's behavior, they would tell him precious little about how a radio works and how it can be fixed unless he possessed prior knowledge of how it works. With language behavior, it is the same, with the present problem being that there is no agreed-upon theory of what language is, let alone how it works in the brain. Thus, the magnificent summary of aphasic disorders by Lhermitte and Gautier[1]—which lists disorders of comprehension as well as disorders of expression, including phonemic disintegration, dysprosody, stereotyped agrammatisms, paraphasia, and the like, each with its own dramatic reality—finds one feeling that some lovely answers are available to a variety of unknown questions. Add to this the fact that disorders of language resulting from brain lesions invariably have, as an integral part of the disease, numerous associated cognitive problems, and the task of identifying the relevance of the observations to a biological understanding of language becomes staggering.

Still, certain facts concerning brain and language have emerged, and in what follows, we will attempt to organize them into a meaningful framework. We will consider our new observations on case P.S., as well as a variety of other clinical and normal data that bear on what we feel are some of the key issues concerning the neural correlates of linguistic processes.

LANGUAGE DEVELOPMENT AND LATERALIZATION

In the vast majority of humans, the left hemisphere is dominant for language. In the remaining small percentage, language develops bilaterally or in the right hemisphere, and the same general regions are thought to be involved in the two half-brains. In particular, the specific areas that seem especially involved are Wernicke's area, the angular gyrus, and the supramarginal gyrus, all located in the posterior temporal–parietal junction, and Broca's area, found at the base of the third frontal convolution (Figure 25).

Detailed knowledge about the microstructure of these areas and how it might relate to language processing is not available. Although anatomical studies have suggested that the planum temporale of the temporal–parietal junction is larger in the left hemisphere of approximately 60% of the population[2], such correlational findings are at present difficult to interpret. The inadequacy of these data is pointed out by the fact that roughly 35% of the remaining population with left-hemisphere language does not have the supposed critical neuroanatomical structure.

There are no data available that bear directly on why language is lateralized, but the indirect evidence points out certain hints. In the first place, it seems that it is really the expressive speech mechanism that demands lateralization. This conclusion is suggested by the original split-brain studies[3,4,5] as well as by our more recent observations on P.S.[28], all of which will be described later. In addition, the main aphasic syndromes resulting from lateralized damage in those subject populations known to have a high incidence of bilateral linguistic representation (sinistrals, anomalous dextrals, and children) are mutism and related expressive dysfunctions[6]. These observations suggest that bilateral linguistic representation primarily insulates these groups from comprehension losses and that the mechanism by which speech is programmed and executed is well lateralized and thus sensitive to unilateral damage.

Further evidence that it is the expressive mechanism that requires lateralization comes from Jones's study of four stutterers[7]. Preoperative sodium amytal testing revealed bilateral speech in all four patients. Following unilateral frontal surgery for problems incidental to stammering, all patients talked normally (no stuttering). Thus, bilateral speech representation seems to be associated with problems in executing vocal control.

Our view of these varied data is that the unilateral represen-

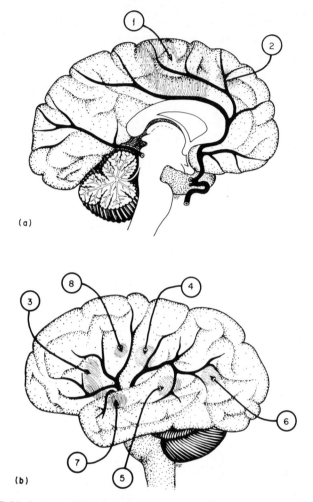

FIGURE 25. Lesions affecting language and speech processes. (1) Area supplied by the anterior cerebral artery. Involves frontoparietal region and the corpus callosum with only transient loss of speech as a result of inclusion of the supplementary motor area. (2) Supplementary motor area of either hemisphere. Stimulation produces arrest of ongoing speech and initiation of repetitive, nonvoluntary vocalization (similar to epileptogenic lesions in the left hemisphere of that area). Lesions result in abnormalities in initiation, continuation, and inhibition of speech. (3) Broca's area, lower part of the premotor zone. Typically produces agrammatism, poor articulation, and abnormal writing of events required for both pronunciation of words and fluent speech. (4) Retrocentral area. Lesions result in

tation of the mechanisms by which speech is programmed and executed provides a final cognitive path through which behavior can be organized and controlled[8,9]. Though both sides of the brain may comprehend and store linguistic information, the unilateral control over speech provides a common point through which the various cognitive activities related to language can be channeled and through which their relative importance is ranked and motor commands are programmed and executed. Therefore, comprehension generally follows where speech goes, though comprehension may clearly set up shop on its own. Whether it normally does in the absence of an acute neuropathological stimulus will be considered later.

Sodium amytal testing has revealed that a small percentage of the population have bilateral speech and are linguistically intact[10]. The extremely small proportion of the human population with bilateral speech attests to nature's antipathy for the model. Nevertheless, an efficiently functioning commissural system could override the deleterious effects of bilateral representation by providing interhemispheric speech synchronization or inhibition of the mechanisms on one side or the other. A similar notion is relevant to the postulated relation between bilateral comprehension and learning disabilities[11-13]. Since many persons who are not learning disabled have bilateral comprehension, it would seem that malfunctioning

---

apraxia of the lips and tongue, lead to disintegration of speech as a whole. (5) Temporal region. Lesions affect the ability to generalize and differentiate phonetic sounds, cause disintegration of phonetic hearing. Lesions usually produce abnormal speech production and poor reading and writing. (6) Temporal–parietal–occipital region. Lesions do not change the external articulated speech but prevent mental integration of separate elements (disturb simultaneous synthesis). Lesions lead to disintegration of rational speech and to disturbance of the understanding of logical, grammatical constructions (semantic aphasia). (7) Bilateral lesion of the temporal lobe, posterior 2/5 of the first and second temporal convolutions, plus posterior half of the island of Reil, extending to the inferior parietal lobe. Shows word deafness, severe motor aphasia, more muteness than paraphasia. (8) Near Broca's in the motor area of the lateral side of the hemisphere. Electrical stimulation results in perseveration of speech. From M. S. Grazzaniga, 1975, Brain mechanisms and behavior, in: M. S. Gazzaniga and C. Blakemore (Eds.), *Handbook of Psychobiology*, New York, Academic Press.

interhemispheric mechanisms could be a critical variable in the disorder.

In spite of the preponderance of left-hemisphere dominance in adults, it appears that linguistic mechanisms emerge bilaterally during early development and only later consolidate in the left hemisphere[6,19]. During this early period, it is as if the child has a split brain[18]. The interhemispheric connections do not fully myelinate, especially those fibers innervating the language areas, until late in development[20]. Until then, each side could be storing engrams, more or less independently, because of a certain ignorance each hemisphere has of what is going on in the other.

It is not known for sure why the left hemisphere emerges as the neuroanatomical site for normal language processing. There are genetic models[14], environmental models[15], extrachromosomal models[16], developmental models emphasizing the relationship between hand and eye[17], and neuroanatomical models[2]. One essential problem with all of these models is the basic fact that either hemisphere is capable of sustaining language development. Moreover, where the final processing occurs seems easily influenced by early brain damage and possibly environmental influences. This fact points out that during development, there is a critical period in which the brain is essentially malleable and language centers can become established on either side. Once this critical period has passed, however, the verbal centers become quite rigid, and subsequent injury finds the organism almost always unable to reestablish language.

Recently, Nottebohm[18] has suggested that the lateralization of human language and the vocal control of bird song might both be attributable to a factor as simple as the rate at which the two sides of the nervous system develop. This view is certainly consonant with the observation that the left pyramidal tract in humans crosses the medullary midline during development prior to the time that the fibers from the right hemisphere cross[35].

The faster (or earlier) development of one half-brain could also be the factor that determines handedness. The more mature hemisphere, like an older sibling, would have the advantage in sensorimotor as well as cognitive development.

In the previous chapter, we developed a model of language lateralization based on the idea that as language becomes left-lateralized, other functions fill in the vacated synaptic space in the right hemisphere. If a lesion of the left side occurs prior to the time that these other functions have acquired space, recovery is seen. Otherwise, it is not.

Recent studies by Nottebohm[18,22] suggest a molecular model that could explain how these shifting and shiftable functions are programmed. In brief, he has shown that the learning of bird song by the young chaffinch can occur only up to the first year of life. If the bird is exposed to the father's song after 12 months, no learning ever occurs. On the other hand, if the young male is castrated, which delays the onset of puberty, the song can be learned up to almost two years.

The essential change that occurs with castration, of course, is the change of blood levels of testosterone, an event that occurs around puberty in humans, which is almost the time that language is "wired out" and is no longer capable of being reestablished. At the biochemical level, it is now known that hormones like testosterone have an enormous effect on neural-cell regulation. Not only is this link exciting at a basic level of neural functioning but it raises intriguing possibilities for a possible molecular approach to rehabilitation.

RIGHT-HEMISPHERE LANGUAGE IN THE LEFT-DOMINANT POPULATION?

Up until the mid-1960s, it was commonly believed that the right hemisphere in man was little involved in language processing. Penfield and others, for example, were able to obtain language phenomena only by stimulating language areas within the left hemisphere[23]. While there were clear exceptions to this general rule, especially in left-handers, the predominant view was that language processing was the business of the left hemisphere.

About that time, a series of tests carried out on Bogen's split-brain patients was reported[5]. In the first set of studies, it was found that the right hemisphere of some patients could comprehend some simple nouns. However, the same patients were totally unable to process verbs and showed little evidence that they could grasp adjectives. Later, another series of linguistic tests were administered, and again it was shown that the right hemisphere was syntactically weak[24]. It seemed to be able to recognize the negative but could not make plurals or comprehend tense and failed on a variety of other tests of syntactical ability. Studies by Levy and Trevarthen revealed that the right hemisphere could not rhyme, and they too came up with a rather meager picture of its language functions[25]. More recently, Zaidel has reported that the right hemisphere in Bogen's patients seems more adept at language[26]. He attributed this increased ability to process language to improved methods of stimulus lateralization, which in effect allows the subject more time to explore the nature of the stimulus.

TABLE 2. Rhyming, Opposite, and Conceptual Matches[a]

	Correct Responses
Rhymes	
Left hemisphere: canoe (new), sky (lie), corn (barn), brook (shook), beet (heat), hall (maul)	4/6
Right Hemisphere: tie (buy), rose (knows), fur (her), knee (pea), stair (care), hoe (dough)	6/6
Opposites	
Left Hemisphere: circle (square), army (navy), cat (dog), bride (groom)	4/4
Right hemisphere: girl (boy), doctor (patient), angel (devil), child (adult)	4/4
Concepts	
Left hemisphere: clock (time), porch (house), devil (hell), crowd (people), shell (turtle), chair (table)	5/6
Right hemisphere: phone (talk), check (bank), nurse (hospital), court (judge), shore (beach), floor (tile)	5/6

[a] In these tests, the first word of each pair shown was lateralized and the word in parentheses was the correct match. Both hemispheres performed well on these tests.

The initial observations on the Wilson series of patients seemed consistent with the earlier findings. The right hemisphere performed poorly on tasks requiring phonemic analysis[27]. The data suggested that while the right hemisphere does understand simple spoken words, it must gain meaning from the whole sound of the word and not from its phonemic elements.

In contrast to all of the other patients examined in both series is case P.S. This patient is truly remarkable from the point of view of linguistic analysis, and it is worth considering some of the right-hemisphere and left-hemisphere language skills that we have noted to date[28]. Within a month after surgery, we observed an incredible range of language skills in both hemispheres, using standard tachistoscopic exposure procedures (Table 2). In brief, the patient was able to rhyme and to recognize opposites and superordinate concepts and was also able to act on printed commands (Table 3).

TABLE 3. Action Verbs and Verbal Commands[a]

		Correct Responses	
		Left Hemisphere	Right Hemisphere
Action verbs:			
Sleeping, laughing, crying, eating, writing, falling, running, drinking, dripping, smoking	(10)	9	10
Verbal commands:			
Hand praxis	(12)	5	5
Finger praxis	(5)	2	3
Whole-body movements	(9)	3	4
Facial and head praxis	(19)	10	12
Engrams for object use	(8)	6	3

[a] Each of the 10 action verbs was visually lateralized to each half-brain. The subject was required to point to the picture that best matched the action described by the verb. Verbal commands or key words in the commands were lateralized, and the subject was required to perform the command. Total trials to each hemisphere are shown in parentheses. The low response rate is accounted for by "no-response" trials and "incorrect-response" trials, both of which may reflect active inhibition or even interference from the "nonseeing" hemisphere (48), as well as failure to comprehend the command or to perceive the word flashed.

Thus, when a word—say, *pie*—was laterally projected to the right hemisphere, the patient would claim that he saw nothing, but then with the left hand, he was able to point to the card that had the picture of a pie on it. With similar procedures, the superordinate classes were managed. For example, when the word *judge* was flashed to the right hemisphere, the patient could choose from a series of cards the most appropriate matching word, which was *trial*. Similarly, P.S. was able to match lateralized "action verbs" to the picture depicting the action. He was also able to carry out printed verbal commands lateralized to either hemisphere. Examples of such commands are "stand," "clap," "laugh," "wink," "wave," and "salute." On other trials, he was told to touch his thumb (or forefinger) to this finger, and the appropriate finger name would then be flashed.

In addition to these right-hemisphere comprehensive skills, which alone distinguished P.S. from all previous split-brain patients, we witnessed expressive capacities in the mute half-brain. A line drawing or a picture of a common object was flashed to the right hemisphere on each of eight trials, and P.S. was asked to spell the name of the item by selecting the appropriate letters from a group and placing them in proper sequence. Irrelevant letters were always included in the group. With little trouble, P.S. spelled *pin, apple, tire, card, bike, leaf, bulb,* and *sheep.*

Most impressive, however, was the ability of the mute half-brain to write with the left hand (Figure 26). It is quite interesting to note that one expressive capacity (writing) can develop and exist in the absence of another (speech), a finding that suggests that each facet of the language process may have its own developmental control mechanism.

This rather startling demonstration of the extent of right-hemisphere language in case P.S. underlines the general rule concerning right-hemisphere language in split-brain patients. In brief, the variation in the amount and kind of language in the mute hemisphere is far greater than the consistency and is most likely a function of the degree and place of early brain damage to the left half-brain. In case P.S., it is known that there was early brain pathology in the left temporal region at the age of 2. The conse-

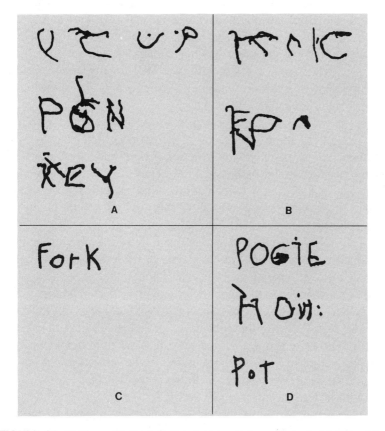

FIGURE 26. Writing with the left and right hands in response to lateralized information. Pictures or line drawings of objects were flashed to one hemisphere or
to the other, and P.S. was asked to write the names of the objects. The left hand,
although clumsy, managed to spell *cup, pen,* and *key,* when these objects were
presented to the right hemisphere (Part A). The left hand was quite incapable of
generating a legible response when a playing card and a fork were presented, on
separate trials, to the left hemisphere (Part B). The right hand was, naturally,
adept at responding to left-hemisphere stimuli (Part C). When the right hand tried
to respond to right-hemisphere stimuli (a light bulb on the first two trials, a cup
on a third), performance deteriorated (Part D).

quence of this lesion would seem to have been to bilateralize the language mechanisms. Similarly, both N.G. and L.B. (the two patients in the Bogen series that can supposedly be shown to have rich right-hemisphere language when tested under prolonged exposure) have been shown to have left temporal seizure foci[29]. In contrast, under standard test conditions, W.J. of the Bogen series, who apparently developed normally through age 30, showed no signs of right-hemisphere language[5,17].

In the more general clinical literature, there are scattered reports suggesting some (though usually minimal) linguistic survival following left hemispherectomy in some right-handed adults with no obvious early brain pathology[30-34]. These few cases, however, which are part of a small population, contrast with the extensive number of patients (global aphasics) who lose all natural language skills following massive left-hemisphere damage.

The right hemisphere has long been viewed as playing an important compensatory role in the recovery from aphasia following left damage[46,47]. However, Hecaen[37] noted that it is generally more plausible to attribute the recovery to remaining left-hemisphere tissue, except in cases of massive damage to the left.

We thus feel that the split-brain and other clinical data provide little positive support for the view that the right hemisphere is normally active in linguistic processing in the left-dominant population. This view is consistent with the recent results of a series of tests administered to normal subjects[36].

These tests made use of the fact that when a word is flashed across the midpoint of the visual field, those letters appearing to the left of center go to the right hemisphere, and those appearing to the right of center go to the left. Thus, if a subject is fixating the midpoint of the word *tyrant,* the first three letters, *tyr-,* go to the right hemisphere, and the last three, *-ant,* go to the left. While it seems reasonable to assume that all six letters must be reassembled before the subject can read the complete word, the experiment was aimed at picking up what the separate hemispheres can do linguistically with the three-letter word segment presented to it before the whole six-letter word is assembled (Figure 27).

In the first experiment, a large list of ordinary six-letter En-

EXPERIMENT I

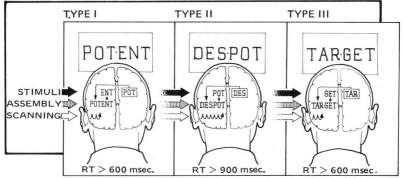

FIGURE 27. Experiment shows the hazards of interpreting clinical data in the framework of the cerebral dynamics of the normal brain. While a variety of clinical studies have suggested that the right hemisphere is capable of simple word discriminations, such as *pot* or *jar,* the reaction-time data under lateralized testing conditions suggest that the right hemisphere passes all word elements over to the left for assembly before processing the entire word. See text for full explanations.

glish words was generated. There were four types: Type 1 words, in which the first but not the last three letters formed a word, for example, *potent;* Type 2 words, in which the last three letters formed a word, for example, *despot;* Type 3 words, in which both three-letter groups formed words, for example, *target;* and Type 4 words, in which neither of the three-letter groups formed words, for example, *foster.* The subject's task in this study was to press a small, vertically mounted lever held between the thumb and the index finger of the right hand if either three-letter segment formed a word. If neither segment formed a word, the subject was required to refrain from pressing.

Again, this procedure meant that when a stimulus of Type 1 (*potent*) was presented, the left hemisphere initially received the nonword portion and the right hemisphere the word portion. The reverse was true when stimuli of Type 2 were flashed. If the subject responded faster to stimuli of Type 2 than to stimuli of Type 1, the result would suggest that the left hemisphere could make a judgment about a part of the word before the entire word was assembled. On the other hand, if the subject responded faster to stimuli of Type 1, in which the three-letter-word segment went to the right hemisphere first, then the result would suggest that the word was assembled in the left hemisphere and scanned from left to right. In other words, if the results took this turn, it would suggest that the right hemisphere does no processing of the information but rather sends it over to the left for assembly and language analysis.

It was found that indeed Type 1 stimuli were responded to approximately 300 msec faster than Type 2 stimuli. The interpretation offered of these findings is that the right hemisphere sends its information over to the left, where the entire word is assembled. After assembly, a scanning process that normally goes from left to right extracts from the three-letter segment the information necessary to make the correct response. These and other studies described in the original report suggest that the right hemisphere, no matter what its potential for linguistic analysis might be in abnormal states, does not, when normal English words are being read, contribute much to the reading process. The studies do not rule out the possibility that the right hemisphere *may* be capable of performing simple linguistic functions, but they do strongly imply that the right-hemisphere linguistic abilities are not heavily relied upon by callosum-intact persons, when reading ordinary prose.

Thus, it would seem that right-hemisphere language in the left-dominant population is only a possibility and clearly is not the rule. Even less likely, however, is the possibility that right-hemisphere language, when it exists in left-dominant persons, is qualitatively different from normal left-hemisphere language[26]. We have found nothing unique about the language capacities present in the right half-brain of P.S., and following early left hemispherectomy, patients can develop normal language skills, though the process is sometimes protracted[21]. We feel that when patients are shown to have unique right-hemisphere language skills, what is being measured is an abnormal and/or arrested development of normal linguistic mechanisms.

LANGUAGE AND PRAXIS

Closely tied to questions concerning the organization of language in the brain are issues associated with the nature of voluntary movement. In the last century, Leipmann suggested that the hemisphere contralateral to the preferred hand is the primary locus of storage of motor engrams for skilled movement[38]. More recently, Geschwind has adopted a similar position[39].

Of particular relevance here are our observations of case P.S. As we described earlier, P.S., who is right-handed, was able to carry out a variety of movements in response to verbal commands directed to his right hemisphere. In addition, he was equally adept with each hemisphere at mimicking finger postures[40] with the contralateral hand, and both hemispheres were poor with the ipsilateral hand. In contrast, while the Bogen patients performed quite similarly to P.S. on the finger-postures test[40], they were unable to carry out right-hemisphere verbal commands[5,17].

These split-brain observations suggest several important points concerning the neurological basis of praxis. In the first place, each separated hemisphere seems to exercise control over the distal musculature of the contralateral but not the ipsilateral hand. Thus, the view that the left hemisphere exercises motor control over both hands is not supported. While it could be argued that early extracallosal damage in split-brain patients institutes a reorganization of motor circuitry so that motor engrams become bilateralized, a recent study of normal subjects suggests otherwise. Lomas and Kimura[41] have shown that the skilled motor activities of the right but not the left hand are interfered with by left-hemisphere activity (talking). This finding is consistent with the split-brain data in that it suggests that the left hemisphere is minimally involved in the control of the motor activities of the left hand.

Second, it would seem that an inability to carry out verbal commands through the right half-brain is more attributable to the absence of linguistic representation than to a lack of motor engrams. In other words, a rich linguistic representation in the right hemisphere, as in P.S., merely allows verbal access to motor skills that are normally present.

These observations allow speculation concerning the the lateralization of handedness and speech. As noted earlier, the left hemisphere may have a developmental edge over the right. As a consequence, the right hand would naturally take the lead early in life. Similarly, the more advanced half-brain would also acquire a more potent linguistic representation. It is easy to see how a "feed-forward" system could be set up that would increase the probability that finely tuned motor skills (including speech) would consolidate in the left.

Whatever advantage the left hemisphere may possess relative to the right in controlling skilled movement, and for whatever reason, the observations on human commissurotomy cases nevertheless suggest that each hemisphere exercises the primary control over the contralateral distal extremities and has relatively poor control over the distal musculature of the ipsilateral extremities. Similar results have been obtained in studies of nonhuman primates[42]. In addition, the observations on P.S. show that in a right-handed patient, each half-brain can have its own store of information of executing and controlling most nondistal motor activities, save for the important exception of speech, for which one half-brain, usually the right, falls short.

ARTIFICIAL AND NATURAL LANGUAGE

Throughout this chapter, we have rather loosely used terms such as *language* and *linguistic* but have done so entirely within the context of normal, human language, by which we mean capacities such as speech production and reception, as well as the reading and writing of speech derivatives. Yet, the fascinating studies of the communicative capacities of chimpanzees, in contrived[43] as well as natural[44] situations, have shown that the cognitive capacities underlying communicative skills are not unique to man in any absolute sense. Of particular relevance here is Premack's success in teaching an artificial language to Sarah[43].

Premack's work with Sarah suggested a possible means of re-habilitating global aphasics—humans with massive lesions of the language-dominant hemisphere that deprive the patient of the ability to speak, comprehend speech, read, and write. Could such patients learn a metalanguage using their intact right half-brain?

In studies carried out with Glass and Premack, it was shown that the totally languageless adult could indeed learn a metalanguage system[45]. In brief, the training program went like this. Preliminary to any language training, a viable social relation was established between the patient and the trainer. This phase was extremely important, for if the motivational setting was inappropriate, no learning would occur. In psychological parlance, if a patient was emotionally flat and showed no preferences, it was impossible to arrange a contingency in which manipulating and learning X would produce desired reward Y. All too frequently, neuropsychological assessment procedures ignore this factor. Tests are designed, norms are established, and the relation all this has to testing a brain-damaged patient, who surely is in a complex, ever-changing motivational state, is just this side of remote.

Consider Mr. J.A., who was a card shark both before and after his stroke. His motivation to learn the system was radically enhanced when the symbols were introduced in the context of a game of cards. Another patient was a carpenter, and so the objects chosen with which to associate words were nuts, bolts, and screws of various shapes and sizes. He was able to judge screws as identical or different with more accuracy than the experimenter. Generally, the reward for correct performance was social; the trainer smiled, expressed pleasure, patted the subject, and so forth. Additional reinforcers, such as food and candy, were sometimes also used. The training procedure and the set of reinforcers, then, were highly individualistic and were geared to the specific patient.

With the use of paper cutout symbols, errorless training procedures were administered in the initial training (Figure 28). For example, in the teaching of "same versus different," two similar objects—say, two apples—were placed on a table in front of the patient. Placed in between was another symbol, a question marker, which came to mean "missing element." The subjects learned to

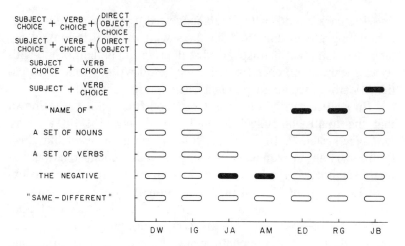

FIGURE 28. As can be seen, the same–different judgment was easily managed by all the aphasics tested. The block boxes indicate only the level of artificial-language training achieved before hospital dismissal. From A. V. Glass, M. S. Gazzaniga, and D. Premack, 1972, Artificial language training in global aphasics, *Neuropsychologia 11:*95–103.

slide the question marker out from between the two test objects and insert in its place the symbol meaning "same." At first, this was the only response allowed. Subsequently, an apple and a screwdriver were placed in front of the patient, and the patient had to remove the question marker and insert the symbol meaning "different." Following this training, the two symbols were both available on each trial, and the subject now had to make the correct response to the two varying "same" or "different" stimuli. When the stimuli used in training were then changed, it was observed that the subjects could use the symbols correctly no matter what test objects were used by the examiner.

These procedures, then, enable one to teach any number of language operations to the global aphasic patient. The "negative," "yes," and "no," the "question," and simple sentences were all successfully taught. Before teaching the sentences, the trainer increased the patient's lexicon by teaching him a few nouns, verbs, and personal names (Figure 29). Each of these words was taught by the association of a symbol with an object, action or agent in the context of a simple social transaction. An object was placed before the patient along with the symbol for the object, and the patient was required to place the symbol on the writing surface, after which he was given the object. The first object was replaced by a second one, along with the word appropriate to it, and the subject was again required to place the name on the writing surface in order to obtain the object. This training too was errorless, as was all training in the initial stages. Learning was assessed as usual by choice trials in which one object was presented along with two words and the subject was required to use the word appropriate to the object.

These results demonstrate that certain cognitive skills can exist independent of natural language. The patients, like chimpanzees, were able to meet the logical and conceptual demands

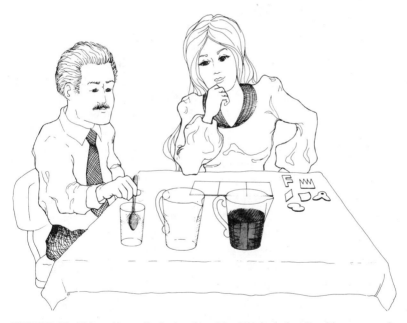

FIGURE 29. Using the methods developed by Premack for the chimpanzee, the global aphasic also learned to ''write'' simple sentences. Here, while the examiner carries out a simple act of stirring the water, the subject is about to arrange the appropriate symbols in a way that effectively says, ''Mike stirs water.''

required to learn the metalanguage. However, it would appear that the cognitive skills of the intact right hemisphere of the global aphasic are probably more like those of a smart chimp than those of a linguistically intact human.

PSYCHOLINGUISTICS AND THE BRAIN SCIENCES

How does brain research illuminate psycholinguistic theory? Some feel that it doesn't and moreover that there is little value in the effort of trying to understand language by studying the brain. If the objective of linguistics is to describe accurately the rules that predict language use in a formal way, then once that is accomplished, the job of the linguist is, in some sense, done. The language behavior of a brain-damaged person, while interesting, may or may not be disrupted in ways that make sense to a formal theory.

For example, the analysis of aphasic patients to date has not isolated syndromes with any specificity that might directly affect a linguistic view of language. There are no reports of patients that have specifically dropped the first, third, or whichever rewrite rule of the sentence. If data from the clinic have anything at all to say about the current linguistic models, it is that the models don't seem to have a reality when aphasic speech is the issue at hand. In one case we studied, the patient was severely aphasic and was totally unable to say "Close the window" or to respond to "Tap the blue block and then the red block." Yet, the patient, a proctological surgeon for 48 years, was able, when asked his opinion of Preparation H, to deliver a five-minute, syntactically correct harangue on why it was crazy to use such products!

Such instances are hard to explain with a simple linguistic model. It would almost seem that the Preparation H answer had been given so many times that it had the status of a punched tape, burped out almost subconsciously. Yet, looked at by itself, it would be material for the linguist to analyze both on the surface and in terms of its deep-structure characteristics. It seems that if such generative processes were working in this instance, they should be working enough to produce the sentence "Close the window."

In addition to most phenomena in aphasia, there are a few common clinical states that have not received proper attention. Patients with dominant-hemisphere damage often suffer from either anomia or dysnomia. This inability to find a noun is never contrasted by observations of patients suffering from *averbia!* What is it about the role of the verb in the language process that makes this part of speech elusive in discrete brain disease? It seems that when verbs do go, the entire language system collapses. The centrality of verbs to the communication process is real. To know a verb is to know a generalization. Whereas an apple is an apple, the verb *pour* can be used in hundreds of contexts. It is of interest to note that in the metalanguage training of aphasics, verbs were difficult to train, whereas symbols for noun-objects were generally learned in one trial.

LANGUAGE AND MEMORY

We feel that the main lessons from the clinic to date also illuminate issues in the way verbal information is organized and stored in the brain. Specifically, when patients with either chronic, steady-state brain damage or patients with transient abnormalities are carefully examined, it becomes apparent that aspects of language are discretely stored in complex interconnecting neural networks so that a lesion breaking a connection between two different storage areas finds the patient unable to use the words and derivative ideas conjunctively. For example, a patient with alexia but without agraphia was recently examined who showed this effect rather dramatically. This syndrome, which is very labile, eventually settles down, and consistent behavior can be observed. In this particular case, the patient had a specific color anomia, which is to say that she could point to a line drawing of a banana, or a frog, or a tree, and when asked what color the items were, she would respond appropriately. However, when asked to state the color of cherries or strawberries, which she could easily discriminate from other line drawings, she was totally and completely unable to say "red." She could pick the color out from a selection of color cards and then call it "reddish, I guess."

The patient was taken through the list several times, and each time she was to name the color of the red fruits, she would say she didn't know. Then she was asked what was the color of a fire engine, and she immediately responded, "Oh, red." How about an old-time schoolhouse? "Red," she shot back. Well, what about cherries? "Gee, I don't know!"

Clearly these data suggest that particular classes of information are stored in particular brain areas. These areas are multiply accessed through specific neural channels, so that accessing red for fruits might be impaired but not red for fire engines. Such observations are truly suggestive of important mental mechanisms, and these will be examined in Chapter 6. For now, however, we leave both memory and language and turn to a not altogether different problem, but one that we will approach somewhat differently, namely, brain and intelligence.

REFERENCES

1. F. Lhermitte and J. C. Gautier, 1969, Aphasia, in: P. J. Vinken and G. W. Bruyn (Eds.), *Handbook of Clinical Neurology,* New York, Wiley.
2. N. Geschwind and W. Levitsky, 1968, Human brain: Left–right symmetries in temporal speech region, *Science 161:*186–187.
3. M. S. Gazzaniga, J. E. Bogen, and R. W. Sperry, 1963, Laterality effects in somesthesis following cerebral commissurotomy in man, *Neuropsychologia 1:*209–215.
4. M. S. Gazzaniga, J. E. Bogen, and R. W. Sperry, 1965, Observations on visual perception after disconnexion of the cerebral hemispheres in man, *Brain 88:*221.
5. M. S. Gazzaniga and R. W. Sperry, 1967, Language after section of the cerebral commissures, *Brain 90:*131–148.
6. J. W. Brown and H. Hecaen, 1976, Lateralization and language representation, *Neurology 26:*183–189.
7. R. K. Jones, 1966, Observations on stammering after localized cerebral injury, *J. Neurol. Neurosurg. Psychiatr. 29:*192–195.

8. M. S. Gazzaniga, 1973, Brain theory and minimal brain dysfunction, *Annals N.Y. Acad. Sci. 205:*89–92.

9. M. S. Gazzaniga, 1974, Cerebral dominance viewed as a decision system, in: S. J. Dimond and D. Beaumont (Eds.), *Hemispheric Functions,* London, Paul Vlek Publishers.

10. B. Milner, C. Branch, and T. Rasmussen, 1966, Evidence for bilateral speech representation in some non-right handers, *Trans. Am. Neurol. Assoc. 91:*306–308.

11. S. T. Orton, 1937, *Reading, Writing, and Speech Problems in Children,* New York, Norton.

12. M. Olson, 1973, Laterality differences in tachistoscopic word recognition in young normal and delayed readers, *Neuropsychologia 11:*3, 393–399.

13. O. L. Zangwill, 1975, Ontogeny of cerebral dominance in man, in: E. H. Lenneberg and E. Lenneberg (Eds.), *Foundations of Language Development,* New York, Academic Press.

14. J. Levy and T. Nagylaki, 1972, A model for the genetics of handedness, *Genetics 72:*117–128.

15. R. L. Collins, 1968, On the inheritance of handedness, *J. Hered. 59:*9–12.

16. M. Corballis and W. Beale, 1976, *The Psychology of Left and Right,* New York, Lawrence Erlbaum Association.

17. M. S. Gazzaniga, 1970, *The Bisected Brain,* New York, Appleton-Century-Crofts.

18. F. Nottebohm, 1977, Origins and mechanisms in the establishment of cerebral dominance, in: M. S. Gazzaniga (Ed.), *Handbook of Behavioral Neurobiology,* New York, Plenum Press.

19. L. S. Basser, 1962, Hemiplegia of early onset and the faculty of speech with special reference to the effects of hemispherectomy, *Brain 85:*28–52.

20. A. LeCours, 1975, Myelogenetic correlates of the development of speech and language, in: E. H. Lenneberg and E. Lenneberg (Eds.), *Foundations of Language Development,* New York, Academic Press.

21. A. Smith and O. Sugar, 1975, Development of above normal language and intelligence 21 years after left hemispherectomy, *Neurology 25:*813–818.

22. F. Nottebohm, 1970, Ontogeny of bird song, *Science 167:*950–956.

23. W. Penfield and L. Robert, 1959, *Speech and Brain-Mechanisms,* Princeton, N.J., Princeton University Press.

24. S. Hillyard and M. S. Gazzaniga, 1971, Language and speech capacity of the right hemisphere, *Neuropsychologia 9:*273–280.

25. J. Levy, 1974, Psychobiological implications of bilateral asymmetry, in: S. J. Dimond and D. G. Beaumont (Eds.), *Hemisphere Function in the Human Brain,* New York, Halsted Press.

26. E. Zaidel and R. W. Sperry, 1975, Unilateral auditory language comprehension on the Token Test following cerebral commissurotomy and hemispherectomy, *Neuropsychologia 15:*1–18.

27. S. P. Springer and M. S. Gazzaniga, 1975, Dichotic testing of partial and complete commissurotomized patients, *Neuropsychologia 13:*345–346.
28. M. S. Gazzaniga, J. E. LeDoux, and D. H. Wilson, 1977, Language, praxis, and the right hemisphere: Clues to some mechanisms of consciousness, *Neurology,* in press.
29. J. E. Bogen and P. J. Vogel, 1974, Neurological status in the long term following complete cerebral commissurotomy, in: F. Michel and B. Schott (Eds.), *Les Syndrômes de disconnexion calleuse chez l'homme,* Lyon, France, Colloque International de Lyon.
30. A. Smith, 1976, Paper presented at the International Neuropsychological Society, Toronto.
31. W. A. Becker, A. Fellman, and H. Rossing, 1974, Neuropsychologische und linguistiche Untersuchungsergernisse bei linksseitiger (Dominant) Hemispherektomie *Fortschr. Med. 92:*525–528.
32. L. A. French, D. R. Johnson, I. A. Brown, and F. B. von Bergen, 1955, Cerebral hemispherectomy for control of intractable convulsive seizures, *J. Neurosurg. 12:*154–164.
33. A. Smith, 1971, Speech and other functions after left (dominant) hemispherectomy, *J. Neurol. Neurosurg. Psychiatr. 29:*467–471.
34. C. W. Burklund, 1972, Cerebral hemisphere function in man: Fact versus tradition, in: W. L. Smith (Ed.), *Drugs, Development, and Cerebral Function,* Springfield, Ill., Charles C Thomas.
35. P. I. Yakolev and P. Rakic, 1966, Patterns of decussation of bulbar pyramids and distribution of pyramidal tracts on two sites of the spinal cord, *Trans. Amer. Neurol. Assoc. 91:*366–367.
36. J. Niederbuhl, M. L. Jouandet, and M. S. Gazzaniga, 1977, Right hemisphere language processing? Not in normals, *Brain Lang.,* in press.
37. H. Hécaen, 1978, Aphasias, in: M. S. Gazzaniga (Ed.), *Handbook of Behavioral Neurobiology,* Vol. 2, New York, Plenum Press, in press.
38. H. Leipmann, 1900, Das Kranicheitsbild der Apraxie auf Grund eines Falles von einseitiger Apraxie, *Monatsschr. Psychiatr. Neurolog. 8:*15–40, 102–132, 182–187.
39. N. Geschwind, 1975, The apraxias, *Am. Sci. 63:*188.
40. M. S. Gazzaniga, J. E. Bogen, and R. W. Sperry, 1967, Dyspraxia following division of the cerebral commissures, *Arch. Neurol. 16:*606–612.
41. J. Lomas and D. Kimura, 1976, Intrahemispheric interactions between speaking and sequential manual activity, *Neuropsychologia 14:*23.
42. S. Brinkman and H. G. J. M. Kuypers, 1973, Cerebral control of contralateral and ipsilateral arm, hand, and finger movements in the split-brain rhesus monkey, *Brain 96:*653–674.
43. D. Premack, 1971, Language in chimpanzees? *Science 172:*808–822.
44. E. Menzel, 1977, Communication of object locations in a group of young chimpanzees, in: D. Hamburg and J. Goodall (Eds.), *Behavior of Great Apes,* New York, Holt, Rinehart, Winston.

45. A. S. Glass, M. S. Gazzaniga, and D. Premack, 1973, Artificial language training in global aphasics, *Neuropsychologia 11:*95–103.
46. K. Kliest, 1933, *Gehirn Pathologie,* Leipzig, Barth.
47. J. M. Neilsen, 1947, *Agnosia, Apraxia, Aphasia: Their Value in Cerebral Localization,* New York, Hoeber.
48. R. Nakamura and M. S. Gazzaniga, 1977, Interhemispheric interference in split-brain monkeys, *Fed. Proc. 32:*367a.

Brain and Intelligence

The problem of brain and intelligence was first approached by Lashley[1]. From his studies, two principles concerning the relation between brain and higher cognitive processes emerged. These were the principles of equipotentiality and mass action. The first suggests that all cortical areas are equally potent in carrying out mental functions, and the second, that cognitive capacity is determined by the total mass of tissue available for information processing.

These principles have dramatically influenced the course of neuropsychology, so much so, in fact, that the field has not yet recovered from their deleterious effects. In this chapter, our goal is first to put mass action and equipotentiality, as Lashley viewed them, forever to rest and then to go on to elucidate the neurological view of intelligence that emerges from studies of split-brain animals and human commissurotomy cases.

CORTICAL EQUIPOTENTIALITY AND INTERHEMISPHERIC DYNAMICS

Traditionally viewed, the notion of cortical equipotentiality readily contrasts with that of cortical specificity. Are cognitive functions dependent upon interchangeable neural mechanisms, or are different cognitive functions carried out by unique patterns of neural circuitry?

On the one hand, the idea of cortical equipotentiality makes little sense when considered in light of the continuing studies of partial and complete commissurotomy in both monkey and man[2-7]. Sectioning of selective commissural sites produces unique and specific deficits in the interhemispheric flow of information. Yet, given such organizational specificity, it is difficult to understand how massive cerebral lesions can leave cognitive processes largely intact, save for certain sensorimotor losses[8-10,25,26]. Such paradoxes are easily resolved when the issue is viewed from the vantage point of interhemispheric dynamics.

Consider the multitude of animal lesion studies that have addressed the problem of localizing the brain mechanisms involved in visual-discrimination learning. While bilaterally symmetric lesions are known to produce clear and specific cognitive deficits, the comparable unilateral lesion has little effect[11,12]. However, if the unilateral lesion is produced in a split-brain animal, the perturbed hemisphere manifests the deficit that is usually seen only after bilateral damage[11,13]. These data suggest a good deal of interhemispheric equipotentiality with regard to homologous areas in opposite hemispheres (excluding, of course, lateralized sensorimotor and cognitive functions, especially in adults) and also highlight the clear absence of cognitive equipotentiality within a hemisphere.

The idea of interhemispheric equipotentiality is dramatically supported by clinical observations of brain-damaged children. Time and again, it has been shown that following the early loss of an entire hemisphere, the remaining half-brain is capable of sustaining cognitive development at high levels[14,15]. Are we really to believe that half of the neocortical mass is sufficient for maintaining higher cortical functioning? This question really takes us to Lashley's other principle, mass action. Let us first summarize here by saying that equipotentiality, as Lashley viewed it, simply does not exist. There is no way that the occipital lobe is going to talk. On the other hand, homologous areas in the two half-brains are, to a large extent, capable of substituting for each other.

MASS ACTION

Lashley felt that the only useful index of cognitive capacity was brain mass. Capacity was thought to depend primarily upon the mass of neural tissue available for information processing. This notion is also the basis of Jerison's theory of the progressive evolution of the brain[16].

These ideas are not by any means wholly accepted by the scientific community. In fact, the current popularity of the anatomical approach in the brain sciences is based on the premise that the critical factor in brain function is the quality of neural connections, not mere tissue quantity.

It thus seems reasonable to approach the problem of brain and intelligence by asking whether the information-processing capacity of the brain is determined by the total mass of tissue available or by the quality of the connections available. As it turns out, the split-brain preparation is ideally suited to an examination of this question.

The idea here is that the single, isolated hemisphere is qualitatively intact, having a nearly complete system of intrahemispheric circuitry, but is quantitatively reduced by half relative to the whole brain. So, if the processing capacity of the half-brain is found to be substantially less than that of the whole brain, then brain mass proves to be the critical factor. Otherwise, the quality of connections reigns. Although various studies have been conducted with this approach and have produced contradictory findings[17-23], when the appropriate control tests are run[24-26], the quality of neural connections proves to be more important than mere quantity as a determinant of cognitive capacity.

How Smart Is the Half-Brain?

The information-processing capacity of the half-brain as opposed to the whole brain has recently been examined in a series of monkey experiments by Richard Nakamura using the nested match-to-sample (NMTS) and the multiple delayed match-to-sample design (MDMTS)[24-26]. These tasks allow for a rather pure measure of information-processing capacity because the discriminative stimuli used can be well trained beforehand, thus minimizing the perceptual demands made on the subjects. This training is particularly important for tests of the processing capacity of animals with sectioned optic chiasms, which the split-brain monkeys have, for the visual apparatus of such animals is significantly impaired relative to that of normals[22].

In the MDMTS task, the subjects were presented with a color (red or green) as the sample stimulus, with the matching colors (red and green) appearing after delays of 0, 2, 6, or 18 sec. This is essentially a short-term memory task.

The results for the MDMTS experiments are shown in Figure 30. As can be seen, normal subjects and chiasm-sectioned splits using one eye or both eyes performed at equivalent levels at all delays. Thus, the data clearly suggest that the short-term memory capacity of the single hemisphere is fully equivalent to that of the whole brain.

The NMTS task requires that the monkey put "on hold" one piece of information while a match-to-sample task is performed. Subsequently, the original piece of information is used in a different match-to-sample task (see Figure 31). For example, first a color stimulus comes on, and then a patterned stimulus is presented. Next, two patterns are presented, one of which must be matched to the original pattern. Finally, two colors come on, one of which matches the original color. Thus, the color-matching problem starts before and finishes after the pattern-matching problem. What makes this task particularly difficult is the fact that across trials the subject is required to retain information about two different samples, and in addition, during each trial, the subject must retain the information necessary to perform the outside task while performing the potentially interfering inside task.

On this task, Nakamura compared the performance of normals, splits, partial splits, and hemispherectomized animals using one eye and both eyes. Figure 32 shows that the only group at a loss was the split group using one eye. Comparison of the performance of hemispherectomized animals and splits using both eyes suggests that the poor performance of the one eye (and one hemisphere) splits did not reflect the processing capacity of the half-brain as opposed to the whole brain. Instead, the data are more consonant with the view that the nonseeing hemisphere of the split actively interferes with the efficient performance of the seeing half-brain. One can prevent interference by removing the poten-

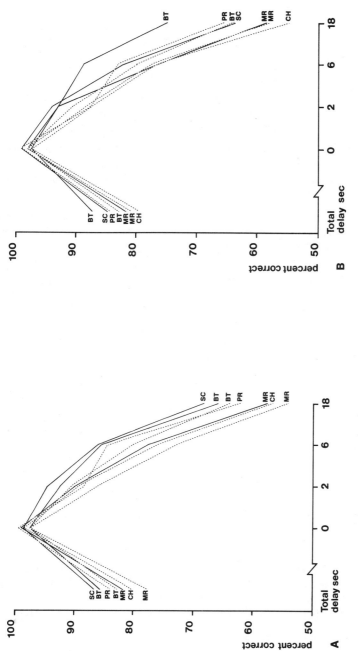

FIGURE 30. Multiple delayed match-to-sample results. Part A depicts the results for the one-eye condition. All animals, whether split (—) or normal (- - -), performed at the same level. The same was true with both eyes open, as shown in Part B. From Nakamura[26].

tially interfering hemisphere, by allowing both half-brains to view the task, or by leaving portions of the interhemispheric pathways intact. Thus, again, we see that the processing capacity of the half-brain is fully equivalent to that of the whole brain.

Observations such as these naturally raise the question of why vertebrates have two cerebral hemispheres. The answer is not likely to be related to cognitive mechanisms but instead to sensorimotor control. After all, primitive vertebrates, whose brains are largely sensorimotor machines, have two hemispheres. In addition, it is primarily sensorimotor losses that result from hemispherectomy in animals, and humans with early hemispherectomy can develop above-average cognitive skills but nevertheless manifest sensorimotor deficits on the effected side[15]. Finally, we must note that the forebrain commissural system, which is largely a means of compensating for the fact that there are two halves of the brain, is primarily concerned with sensorimotor functions (see Chapter 2).

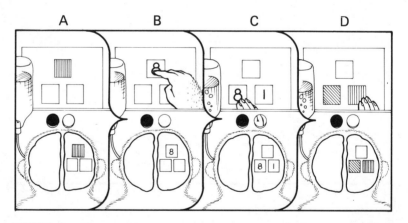

FIGURE 31. The nested match-to-sample task. A split-brain monkey looks through the right eye-hole (unfilled circle). A pattern comes on and is stored (A). Then a number comes on (B). The subject then has to match to the previous number (C). Finally, two patterns come on (D), and the subject has to match to the original pattern seen in A. Thus, the pattern task starts before and ends after the number match. From Nakamura[26].

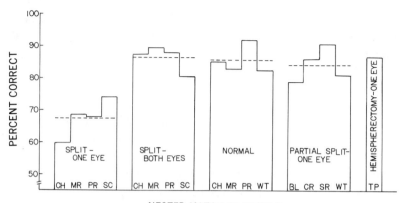

NESTED MATCH TO SAMPLE

FIGURE 32. Nested match-to-sample results. Normal, split, partially split, and hemispherectomized monkeys were tested under monocular and binocular exposure conditions. Only the monocular splits were disadvantaged. However, comparison of the performance of the hemispherectomized and normal animals suggests that the deficit of the split animals using one eye was not a reflection of the processing deficiency of the half-brain but instead represented interference from the nonseeing hemisphere (see text). From Nakamura[26].

Cognitive Cost of Commissurotomy

The implication of the Nakamura data is that the cognitive cost of commissurotomy is minimal, at least when both half-brains are allowed to participate. While these results are consistent with the earlier reports on the Bogen patients, in which it was suggested that there were no obvious psychological deficits unattributable to extrasurgical pathology[27,28], a more recent report by Zaidel and Sperry[29] suggests that commissurotomy patients suffer severe and lasting deficits in information-processing capacity, particularly short-term memory capacity, when tested under conditions of free (unlateralized) vision. This conclusion, however, was based solely on postoperative test scores, which were compared with published scores obtained by normal and unoperated epileptic subjects.

We had the opportunity to examine the cognitive effects of commissure sectioning by running preoperative control tests on case D.H. This is the first recorded commissurotomy case in which an extensive evaluation of the cognitive status of the patient was obtained preoperatively. We used traditional tests (so that our results would be comparable to those of Zaidal and Sperry), as well as a group of relatively new and heuristically sophisticated information-processing tasks, such as the hypothesis task[31], the Buschke selective-reminding-in-free-recall task[32], and the digit-span experimental-memory task. For illustrative purposes, we present the results of two standardized tests (the Wechsler Memory Scale and the Wechsler Adult Intelligence Scale, or WAIS) and one experimental task (the hypothesis task). Regardless, however, the pattern of results on all tests was essentially the same.

In Figure 33, the results of the Wechsler Memory Scale[33] are presented. As can be seen, there was certainly no indication of postoperative memory deficit, nor was there any hint that D.H. was deficient relative to the general population. These findings are consistent with the results of the administration of the WAIS (Table 4).

The hypothesis task, which has evolved out of the theoretical work of Levine[31], is a complex learning task in which the subject is faced with a rapidly changing multidimensional-stimulus situation. His objective is to discover the correct aspect of the stimulus complex by testing various hypotheses. This difficult task substantially taxes short-term memory and other processing skills.

Stimulus slides were rear-projected onto a viewing screen in front of D.H. Each slide contained two seven-dimensional stimuli. The seven dimensions are illustrated in Figure 34. It should be apparent that the two stimuli in Figure 34 are complementary. That

TABLE 4. Preoperative and Postoperative Scores Obtained by D.H. on the Wechsler Adult Intelligence Scale (WAIS)[a]

	Preoperative	Postoperative
Verbal	97	113
Performance	86	90
Full scale	92	103

[a]Different forms of the WAIS were used for the pre- and postoperative testing.

is, if a border on the right stimulus is a circle, then the border on the left must be a square. Similarly, if the letter *A* appears on the left, then the letter *T* must appear on the right. Thus, each of the seven dimensions is composed of two complementary stimulus values, one of which appears in the left stimulus pattern, the other in the right.

A problem consisted of 12 trials. On each trial, D.H. examined one slide containing the complementary seven-dimensional stimuli for several seconds. This was not a lateralized test. The slides were constructed so that when placed in proper sequence, values from either three or four of the seven dimensions changed sides on every trial. The values changed sides in accordance with the rules of internal orthogonality[31]. These rules ensured that each successive slide was a logical outcome of the slide preceding it.

For each problem, only one of the 14 stimulus features was correct (as predetermined by the experimenter). Before the trial,

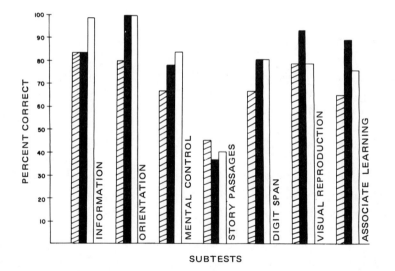

FIGURE 33. Performance of D.H. on the Wechsler Memory Scale. Postoperative performance (■) was compared with preoperative performance (▨) and standardized norms (□). There was no evidence of a postoperative memory deficit. From LeDoux *et al.*[30].

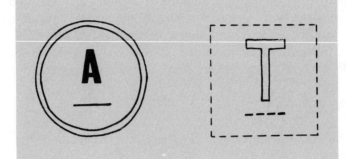

FIGURE 34. Hypothesis-task stimuli: a sample slide. This figure illustrates the complementary seven-dimensional stimuli. The seven dimensions are letter name, letter size, letter color, border shape, border texture, number of borders, and underline texture. Thus, the left stimulus contains the following values: *A*, small, black, circle, solid border, two borders, and solid underline. The complementary values of the right stimulus include *T*, large, white, square, dashed border, one border, and dashed underline. From LeDoux *et al.*[30].

D.H. picked the stimulus feature that he thought was correct, and he verbally stated it. The slide then came on, and he said left or right, depending on which side the feature that he had selected was on. He was then told whether his choice of left or right was correct but was given no information concerning his stimulus choice. His objective was to use this partial feedback to crack the coding scheme of the task. An example of perfect hypothesis testing in shown in Figure 35.

D.H.'s preoperative and postoperative performance is depicted in Figure 36. By all objective standards, D.H.'s postoperative performance was superior to his preoperative performance on this complex information-processing task.

The results of these standardized and experimental information-processing tests demonstrate that callosal sectioning per se does not produce cognitive deficits. Performance did not drop postoperatively and, in fact, seemed to improve some. Moreover, neither preoperative nor postoperative performance was subnormal.

The discrepancy between these data and the observations on

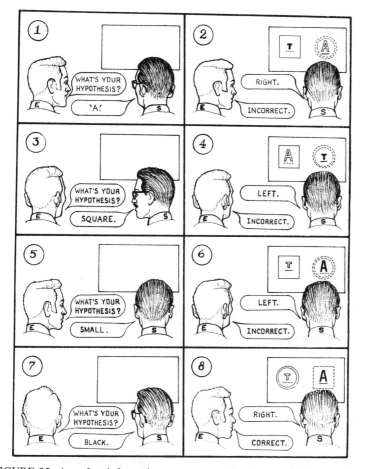

FIGURE 35. A perfect information processor performing on the hypothesis task. Perfect processing during the information trials of a problem is depicted here. Subject and Experimenter are indicated by letters on their collars. The top caption belongs to the first speaker in the frame. Each row (two frames) represents one complete trial. The subject guesses "blindly" from a set of 14 hypotheses on Trial 1 prior to seeing the first stimulus of the problem. Feedback on Trial 1 allows the perfect-processing subject to "focus" in on the seven values in the left stimulus, as he was told that his choice of the right stimulus was incorrect. Thus, on Trial 2, the subject selects from small, black, T, dashed underline, solid, square, and single border. Following feedback on Trial 2, the subject eliminates those values that were on the right on Trial 1 and on the left on Trial 2, leaving small, black, and T as possible solutions. On Trial 3, small and T are eliminated, leaving black as the correct hypothesis (H +). From LeDoux et al.[30]

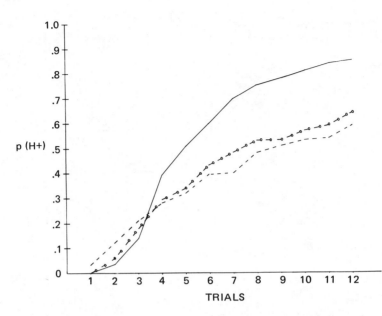

FIGURE 36. Hypothesis task results. Curve 1 represents the first preoperative block (---) of 64 problems, and Curve 2 represents the second block (-o-o-o). Postoperative performance (—) is depicted in Curve 3. D.H. was clearly a more efficient hypothesis-tester postoperatively. From LeDoux et al.[30].

the Bogen patients is worth considering. Zaidel and Sperry were unable to establish preoperative baselines and thus had to rely on published control data. Such comparisons are naturally risky when such a small sample is involved. In contrast, although our data are based on a single subject, the controlled (pre-op, post-op) comparisons unequivocally argue against the notion that the callosum is a critical structure in mnemonic processing. In addition, it should be noted that the WAIS scores of the Bogen patients were in general in the low normal to subnormal range, as were the memory-test scores. The fact that D.H. was clearly "normal" on these standardized tests suggests that other factors besides callosal sectioning might be at the core of the deficient performance of the other patients. One important consideration is extracallosal pathology. Each patient comes into surgery with a unique neurological history. D.H., for example, in addition to callosotomy, earlier underwent decompression of the right temporal pole, and his seizure foci were found to be diffusely spread over the right hemisphere prior to callosal sectioning. In contrast, four of the Bogen patients had bilateral seizure foci (involving the temporal lobe in at least three and possibly all four cases), and two others had left temporal foci[37]. Clearly, with such extensive temporal-lobe pathology in these patients, only pre- and postoperative comparisons on each patient could have provided valid information concerning the effects of callosal sectioning on memory and other cognitive processes.

These observations on human commissurotomy cases and split-brain monkeys leave us on the whole doubting whether there are cognitive costs to commissure sectioning per se. In addition, the data suggest that information-processing cognitive capacity is more dependent upon the quality of neural connections than upon the mass of neural tissue available. In other words, intelligence, cognitive capacity, and the like really reflect the complexities of intrahemispheric mechanisms and thus are only indirectly dependent upon the interhemispheric integration made possible by the great cerebral commissures. Why this is the case is suggested by the following consideration of the relationship between neural circuitry and higher cognitive functioning.

The Neurology of Intelligence

Certain jawless fish living in the depth and darkness of the ocean floor are dependent upon touch receptors for locating food. These receptors detect potential food items and initiate the motor programs necessary for bringing the mouth into contact with the item. Once the item is in the mouth, a different class of receptors actually scrutinize the palatability of the substance. If it passes this test, the item is swallowed. Otherwise, it is regurgitated. However, should the touch receptors again come into contact with the regurgitated substance, the item is retested in the mouth and again regurgitated. This process could continue indefinitely, for the sensory system that detects potential food is not in communication with the system that tests palatability.

The progressive evolution of the brain and intelligence is typified by an increasing capacity for intersensory communication. This notion is supported both anatomically and behaviorally[34,35] and is at the heart of several contemporary biological models of intelligence[16,35]. However, while a variety of creatures seem to have the capacity for biologically appropriate intersensory association, true sensory–sensory association is largely a primate achievement. Although such associations are readily accomplished by either the verbal or the nonverbal hemisphere in man[28], nonhuman primates find such problems difficult, though not impossible[28,36]. Yet, such capacities seem to be totally lacking in nonprimates[35].

The forebrain commissural system, with its massive network of largely homotopic fibers, is a within-modality rather than a between-modality communication channel. Although homotopic associations are sufficient and even necessary for maintaining the flow of highly specified neural codes between the hemispheres (see Chapter 2), they are minimally involved in heterotopic, intersensory integration. To the extent that cross-modality processing reflects higher cognitive skills, it is obvious why callosal sectioning fails to produce striking deficits in intellectual capacities.

While the capacity for sensory–sensory integration does seem to provide a means of making gross statements about the cognitive capacities of different groups of animals, it is nevertheless a worthless indicator of individual differences. As all neurologically intact humans are able to feel an object and subsequently recognize it by sight, such tests are of little use in discriminating between different humans. The problem here is that sensory–sensory integration abilities are not synonymous with "higher intelligence" but are merely one index of the evolved neural substrate that maintains human intelligence and distinguishes it from fish intelligence. More accurately, the evolution of brain and intelligence is characterized by an increase in the complexity of connection not just between sensory systems but in the overall pattern of intrahemispheric brain organization. Such complexities surely reflect—and, in fact, probably determine—the nature of individual differences and are really at the heart of human nature and its characteristic flexibility.

All of this is not to undercut the role of interhemispheric mechanisms in maintaining integrated mental functioning. While callosal sectioning does not seem to alter substantially the raw processing capacity of the brain, we cannot be so sure of its effects on the adaptive behavior (which ultimately reflects sensorimotor efficiency) of the whole organism in the real world. The sensory input to each hemisphere is, after all, substantially reduced without the commissural sensory window (see Chapter 2). There is also the suggestion of long-term motor coordination deficits in split-brain patients[38,39]. In addition, it is unlikely that the two independent mental systems (each with its own sensory input, processing and storage mechanisms, and motor output) would maintain equivalent attentional and motivational states over an extended period. It is only by way of an active interhemispheric communication system that the sensory input to each potentially independent half-brain is maximized, the processing and output mechanisms are coordinated, and, as a result, the adaptive capacity of the integrated organism is maintained at its fullest potential.

REFERENCES

1. K. Lashley, 1950, In search of the engram, *Symposia of the Society for Experimental Biology 4:*454–482.
2. M. S. Gazzaniga, 1966, Interhemispheric communication of visual learning, *Neuropsychologia 4:*183–189.
3. P. Black and R. E. Myers, 1964, Visual functions of the forebrain commissures in the chimpanzee, *Science 146:*799–800.
4. M. V. Sullivan and C. R. Hamilton, 1972, Interocular transfer of reversed and nonreversed discriminations via the anterior commissure in monkeys, *Physiol. Behav. 10:*355–359.
5. M. S. Gazzaniga and H. Freedman, 1973, Observations on visual process after posterior callosal section, *Neurology 23:*1126–1130.
6. M. S. Gazzaniga, G. L. Risse, S. P. Springer, E. Clark, and D. H. Wilson, 1975, Psychologic and neurologic consequences of partial and complete cerebral commissurotomy, *Neurology 25:*10–15.
7. G. L. Risse, J. E. LeDoux, S. P. Springer, D. H. Wilson, and M. S. Gazzaniga, 1977, The anterior commissure in man: Functional variation in a multisensory system, *Neuropsychologia,* in press.

8. A. Smith and C. W. Burklund, 1966, Dominant hemispherectomy, *Science* *153:*1280.

9. A. Smith, 1969, Non-dominant hemispherectomy, *Neurology 19:*442.

10. R. Nakamura and M. S. Gazzaniga, 1975, Comparative aspects of short-term memory mechanisms, in: J. A. Deutsch and D. Deutsch (Eds.), *Short-Term Memory,* New York, Academic Press.

11. M. Mishkin, 1965, Visual mechanisms beyond the striate cortex, in: R. W. Russel (Ed.), *Frontiers in Physiological Psychology,* New York, Academic Press.

12. R. Thompson, 1965, Centrencephalic theory and interhemispheric transfer of visual habits, *Psychol. Rev. 72:*385–398.

13. M. S. Gazzaniga, 1966, Interhemispheric communication of visual learning, *Neuropsychologia 4:* 183–189.

14. L. S. Basser, 1962, Hemiplegia of early onset and the faculty of speech with special reference to the effects of hemispherectomy, *Brain 85:*427–460.

15. A. Smith and O. Sugar, 1975, Development of above normal language and intelligence 21 years after left hemispherectomy, *Neurology 25:*813–818.

16. H. J. Jerison, 1973, *Evolution of the Brain and Intelligence,* New York, Academic Press.

17. J. A. Sechzer, 1970, Prolonged learning and split-brain cats, *Science 169:*889–892.

18. T. H. Meikle and J. A. Sechzer, 1960, Interocular transfer of brightness discrimination in split-brain cats, *Science 132:*734–735.

19. T. H. Meikle, 1964, Failure of interocular transfer of brightness discrimination in split-brain cats, *Science 132:*734–735.

20. T. J. Voneida and J. S. Robinson, 1971, Visual processing in the split-brain cat: One versus two hemispheres, *Exp. Neurol. 33:*420–431.

21. C. R. Butler, 1968, A memory-record for visual discrimination habits produced in both cerebral hemispheres of monkeys when only one hemisphere has received direct visual information, *Brain Res. 10:*152–167.

22. G. Berlucchi, 1974, Some features of interhemispheric communication of visual information in brain damaged cats and normal humans, in: F. Michel and B. Schott (Eds.), *Les syndrômes de disconnexion calleuse chez l'homme,* Lyon, France, Colloque International de Lyon.

23. C. R. Hamilton, 1976, Investigations of perceptual and mnemonic lateralization in monkeys, in: S. Harnad (Ed.), *Lateralization in the Nervous System,* New York, Academic Press.

24. R. Nakamura and M. S. Gazzaniga, 1977, Processing capacities following commissurotomy in the monkey, *Exp. Neurol. 56:*323–333.

25. R. Nakamura and M. S. Gazzaniga, 1977, Information processing in the monkey following hemispherectomy, *Exp. Neurol.,* submitted.

26. R. Nakamura, 1976, Cerebral information processing in the monkey: One versus two hemispheres, unpublished doctoral thesis, SUNY at Stony Brook, New York.

27. M. S. Gazzaniga, J. E. Bogen, and R. W. Sperry, 1965, Observations on visual perception after disconnexion of the cerebral hemispheres in man, *Brain* 88:221.
28. M. S. Gazzaniga, 1970, *The Bisected Brain,* New York, Appleton-Century-Crofts.
29. D. Zaidel and R. W. Sperry, 1974, Memory impairment after commissurotomy in man, *Brain* 97:263–272.
30. J. E. LeDoux, G. L. Risse, S. P. Springer, D. H. Wilson, and M. S. Gazzaniga, 1977, Cognition and commissurotomy, *Brain* 100:87–104.
31. M. Levine, 1969, Neo-noncontinuity theory, in: G. Bower and J. T. Spence (Eds.), *The Psychology of Learning and Motivation,* Vol. 3, New York, Academic Press.
32. H. Buschke, 1973, Selective reminding for analysis of memory and learning, *J. Verb. Learn. Behav.* 12:543–550.
33. D. Wechsler, 1945, A standardized memory scale for clinical use, *J. Psychol.* 19:87–95.
34. E. G. Jones and T. P. S. Powell, 1970, An anatomical study of converging sensory pathways within the cerebral cortex of the monkey, *Brain* 93:793–820.
35. N. Geschwind, 1965, Disconnexion syndromes in animals and man, *Brain* 88:237–294, 585–644.
36. R. K. Davenport, C. M. Rogers, and I. S. Russell, 1975, Cross-modal perception in apes, *Neuropsychologia* 13:229–235.
37. J. E. Bogen and P. J. Vogel, 1974, Neurological status in the long term following complete cerebral commissurotomy, in: F. Michel and B. Schott (Eds.), *Les syndrômes de disconnexion calleuse chez l'homme,* Lyon, France, Colloque International de Lyon.
38. B. F. B. Preilowski, 1972, Possible contribution of the anterior forebrain commissures to bilateral motor coordination, *Neuropsychologia* 10:267–277.
39. D. Zaidel and R. W. Sperry, 1977, Long term motor coordination problems following cerebral commissurotomy, *Neuropsychologia* 15:193–204.

Brain, Imagery, and Memory

While "imagery" has a long history in the study of the mind, going back at least to David Hume in the 18th century, who viewed images as weak sensations [1], the topic is currently at the forefront of that domain of experimental science known as *cognitive psychology*. Although the current popularity of imagery research has resulted in the delineation of certain psychological properties of the image [2-4], little effort has been extended toward elucidating the brain mechanisms involved. Yet, progress in this area would undoubtedly help to specify clearly the nature of the image. Furthermore, an understanding of the neural mechanisms of imagery would have wide-ranging implications for bridging the gap between mind and brain, for imagery is truly a "mental" function. We feel that our continuing studies of the Wilson patients have provided some insights into the neuropsychological nature of mental imagery. The observations to be described were made in conjunction with Dr. Gail Risse [22].

HOW VISUAL IS VISUAL IMAGERY?

Case J.Kn. provided the opportunity for examining one of the basic questions concerning the nature of the visual image. Is the visual image really visual? Alternatively, does visual imagery involve the same neural circuitry as visual sensations and perceptions? Our way of testing this notion was to see if J.Kn.'s intact anterior commissure, which clearly transferred visual sensations between his hemispheres (see Chapter 2), could also transfer visual images. In carrying out this test, we capitalized upon the fact that as a consequence of callosal sectioning, J.Kn. was tactually split.

A common object was placed, out of sight, in J.Kn.'s right hand, and he was instructed to palpate the object carefully and to "make a picture" of it in his mind. When he indicated that he could "see" the object, his left hand was placed in a box and he was asked to find the object. In trial after trial, he was unable to retrieve the imagined object. Yet, if a picture of the object was flashed to his left hemisphere, he was able to find it with his left hand. This response required that the visual input to the left hemisphere cross over to the right through the anterior commissure. Thus, while visual sensory information flows through the anterior commissure, visual images seem not to. So, on the neural level, the visual image seems to be distinct from visual sensory-perceptual experience.

While a negative finding should always be viewed with suspicion, recent observations on D.S. are consistent with the view that visual experience and visual imagery utilize distinct patterns of neural circuitry. Prior to surgery, D.S. was tested on a word-pair memory task. The word pairs were first read to him. Subsequently, the first word of the pair was read, and he was to provide the matching word. He recalled 2 of 10. However, when a different list of word pairs was read and D.S. was given the instruction to image a picture involving the two words (like a "cat" on an "elephant's" back), he recalled 8 of 10. This pattern is quite normal. Postoperatively, however, he recalled 2 of 10 without imagery and 2 of 10 with imagery.

Consider D.S.'s unique neurosurgical history. At the age of 4, he was hospitalized for the removal of a malignant tumor of the left prefrontal cortex. As a consequence of frequent and severe seizure activity localized to the region of scar tissue from the earlier removal, his frontal callosal connections were severed at age 24.

Thus, the implication here is that the preoperative performance on the word-pair task was sustained primarily by the right frontal lobe and its commissural connections to the undamaged areas of the left hemisphere. Section of only the anterior callosal connections presumably left the capacity to image intact but isolated from the verbal mechanisms of the left hemisphere, which surely play a critical role in associating word pairs. Other patients with no frontal damage but complete collosal sections perform normally on the task under both the imagery and the no-imagery conditions, which indicates that the imagery effect can be accomplished within the verbal half-brain.

These observations suggest the possibility that the frontal cortex plays a crucial role in imagery phenomena. The flattened affect and the inability to plan ahead typically noted in patients with frontal-lobe disease might well be related to a loss of the capacity to fantasize and imagine what is going to happen next.

As cell populations in the frontal cortex are not generally thought of as being directly involved in visual perception, the data suggest, as before, that visual imagery is mediated by neural mechanisms that are distinct from the mechanisms of true visual experience. Observations such as these do not fit well within the theoretical framework that has emerged to explain imagery phenomena. It is generally believed that imagery is intimately related to the process of perception, the key difference being that imagery takes place in the absence of the stimulus being perceived[5-7]. This view largely reflects the lasting influence of the British empiricists on the neurological and psychological sciences. These philosophers treated all mental phenomena as derivatives of sensory experience, with images being weak sensations. Thus, the classical view in neurology came to be that the visual cortex is critically involved in visual imagery[25]. Hebb has suggested that imagery might be the result of excitation of complex and hypercomplex cells (à la Hubel and Weisel) in the absence of sensory excitation of simple cells[26]. While such notions are interesting, our data suggest a much more mentalistic view of imagery and other mechanisms of the mind.

It is as if mental life is transacted in codes that transcend perceptual experience on the neural level. This is not to suggest, however, that mental codes are modality-nonspecific, for various experiments suggest otherwise[2,5-7]. Instead, while mental processes may involve modality-specific circuitry, that circuitry would seem to be distinct from the circuitry that mediates the perception of environmental information. Indeed, it should not be too surprising if the neural mechanisms that have evolved for transacting business with the external world (i.e. perceptual-motor mechanisms) are not the mechanisms by which we conduct our mental life.

MEMORY

A primary objective in neuroscience is to establish how and through what processes information is stored in the central nervous system. Memory is rarely both the necessary and the sufficient condition for conscious experience, but it is invariably a necessary and key condition. Yet the long-standing questions of how and where information is stored and by what brain mechanisms it is accessed are as elusive today as ever before, at the molecular level as much as at the psychological level.

To begin with, most of us vault over the initial problem that must be solved by a viable model of memory, namely, how does the organism recognize either internally or externally generated stimuli and put them into a form that can be used in a relevant memory search? The trend is to bypass such questions, to proceed by accepting the notion that there is an inherent organization in information-storage systems, and then to go on to study differences in organizational properties through reaction time, recognition, and recall tasks at the experimental-psychological level and through brain lesions, electrical stimulation, pharmacological manipulations, and the like at the physiological level. While these studies are sometimes intriguing, they rarely leave us with any feeling for how the memory-storage and -retrieval system actually works.

In the following, our aim will be to focus on how a variety of split-brain and other clinical studies have contributed to present understanding of the physical basis of information storage. While some problems and data from animals will be reviewed that highlight what we consider to be facts on the subject of learning and memory, it is our guess that real insights into the biology of memory can be best obtained at this time by a consideration of clinical data. The thrust of the evidence to be described is that the brain has a variety of ways to encode and store information and that a given information-storage system in the brain is not necessarily accessible to every other network of stored information. These data have dramatic implications for traditional interpretations of the mechanisms of memory.

Basic Issues in Learning and Memory: Errors, Rewards, and Motives

After the dramatic breakdown in the interhemispheric transfer of discrimination learning on visual and tactile problems had been shown—a breakdown that underlined the importance of the cortical commissural system in the intercortical exchange of information—little else was forthcoming from the split-brain literature on what the technique teaches about learning and memory per se. Experiments to date indicate only that if the corpus callosum is intact during training, there is usually evidence that a bilateral engram is formed. While there are good indications that complex codes are transmitted through the commissures in animals and man, there is no evidence for the transfer of an engram per se (see Chapter 2).

Nonetheless, it is our contention that the split brain is one of the most exciting preparations that can be used to get at questions of more general interest in the understanding of learning and memory. Consider the series of monkey studies carried out by David Johnson[8,9]. A pattern discrimination was taught to one separated hemisphere. The animal was overtrained and consequently performed perfectly on the task. The eye connected to the naive hemisphere was then exposed and was allowed to observe the errorless performance of the trained half-brain for 40 trials (see Figure 37). The researcher then probed the naive hemisphere for knowledge of the problem by giving trials to it alone, and it performed well.

With errors not a necessary condition for learning, it was then asked whether the organism needs a "reward." So in another set

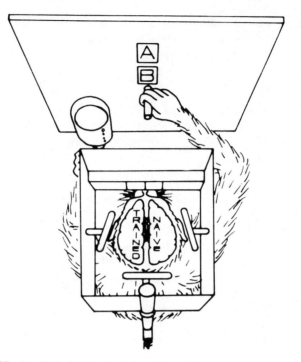

FIGURE 37. A split-brain monkey observing a visual discrimination through a specially designed training apparatus that allows for the separate or combined projection of visual information to each eye. Here, a naive hemisphere is free to observe the errorless performance of a trained hemisphere. From Gazzaniga[21].

of animals, a discrimination was trained to one hemisphere while the other, through the use of polaroid filters[10], saw a blank field. The reward schedule was then advanced so that the animal was rewarded only on every other trial. This schedule did not prove disruptive in any way. Then, on nonrewarded trials, the naive hemisphere was allowed to see the visual discrimination. The question was, Could it learn by observing the trained hemisphere perform the task perfectly in the absence of reward? What was found was that the normal response pattern was totally disrupted, and no learning took place after two experimental sessions. In a subsequent experiment[11], however, when the number of days on which the nonrewarded observational trials were presented was extended, learning did occur. This outcome leaves us with one more—or, more accurately, one less—essential condition needed for discrimination learning to occur, namely, the presence of a primary reward.

These data raise the question of what role reward plays in learning and memory. One interpretation is that its importance lies in engaging the organism to attend to a particular task and that it plays little or no role in the brain mechanisms involved in information storage. Put differently, reward merely signals the organism that a particular event is to be stored, but the storage process itself is not dependent upon the brain mechanisms underlying reward. What is critical for information storage is pure, simple contiguity. Rewards are thus reduced to motives.

This, of course, is not to undercut the importance of rewards as motives. Some learning theories explicitly acknowledge that without motivation there is no learning[12], which raises the possibility that in animal lesion studies, group differences in learning capacity largely reflect differential motivational levels. Further, one often wonders whether the difference in learning ability of the two hemispheres commonly seen in splits[13] reflects differences in motivation—possibly brought about by subcortical brain damage incidentally incurred during split-brain surgery, for unilateral hypothalamic lesions produce striking differences in the eating rates of the two hemispheres of split monkeys[14,15] (see Figure 38). The implication here for variations in normative data on cognitive tasks is, alas, that these variations may largely reflect motivational variables.

The role of reward needs to be considered in more detail. We subscribe to Premack's view that reinforcement is relative and is a function of response probabilities[16]. Thus, Stimulus A can reinforce Stimulus B only if the organism has a higher probability of responding to A than to B. With this view, one can escape from Skinner's tautological approach, in which a reinforcer is what is discovered to be reinforcing[17]. Now, before saying that A is rewarding, we separately and independently measure the probability

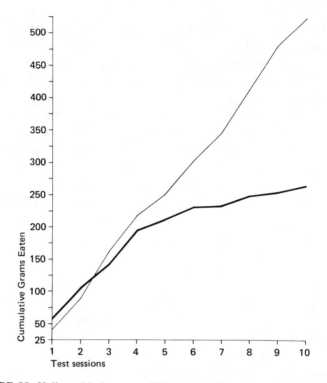

FIGURE 38. Unilateral lesions can differentially affect the motivational state of the separated hemispheres. The right cerebrum has a discrete hypothalamic lesion but also a considerable amount of other brain damage, which disallows conclusions on the contribution of the hypothalamus alone. The main point here is that following cerebral commissurotomy alone, the split-brain animal shows a striking difference in eating behavior as a function of eye use. Left eye (—), right eye (—). From Gibson [15].

that an animal will choose A over B. If the probability is greater than 0.5, we can accurately predict that receiving A contingent on doing B will increase the probability of doing B.

The importance of viewing these processes in relative terms is, it seems to us, especially critical when one is trying to understand the underlying physiology. The Skinnerian view—that an organism has a repertoire of responses and that a particular one comes to the fore only as a result of external contingencies—strikes us as static and passive. The Premack view is more organic in that it sees the organism as actively and continuously assigning values to all stimuli and in that it views response probabilities, which are generated by the organism, as key regulators of behavior.

Yet, curiously, it is the static Skinnerian view that has dominated physiological thinking. How many times have we heard about reward centers that interact with cognitive cortical centers? The view has been that it is reward that freezes or etches into the brain the particular information that an organism is processing. All we have to do is locate the reward center and trace its connections to the higher centers, and we shall then know the primary neural circuits of behavior—of learning and memory. Experiments that contradict this paradigm go unnoticed. For example, it has been shown that a rat with an electrode in a reward center increases its rate of self-stimulation in order to gain the opportunity to run. In other words, running is rewarding the reward center.

In recent work, this basic insight has been applied in a more physiological setting[18]. Lesions in the lateral hypothalamus predictably rendered rats adipsic. They showed, postoperatively, essentially no probability of drinking but did run for approximately 150 sec in 30 min. When the two events were made contingent, so that in order to run the rats had to drink, drinking commenced immediately (Figure 39).

These data taken together serve as a fair warning not to take too literally the idea that memory and mental processing systems can be located in the brain in a simple sense. If one changes the external contingencies of training before or after a brain lesion, seemingly obvious and reliable neurobehavioral symptoms indicating specificity of function tend to disappear. This response leaves the problem of localization of function as mercurial as ever. On the positive side, however, these data suggest that as the motivational state changes, access to innate or learned behavioral patterns, which we think are multiply represented in the brains of both animals and men, is allowed expression. This brings us to what we mean by the multiple representation of the engram.

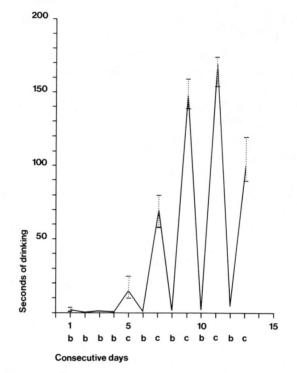

FIGURE 39. Rats with lateral hypothalamic lesions did not drink on baseline (b) days when free access to drinking and running was allowed. They did run, however, and when the two behaviors were made contingent (c), drinking immediately commenced. When the contingency was removed, drinking behavior again returned to a low level. From Gazzaniga *et al.*[18].

Multiple Neural Coding

A frequent assumption in the study of memory is that information is stored in only one fashion: there is "a" brain mechanism for the storage of information, and this same mechanism is used in all storage processes.

An alternative and more dynamic view of how the brain manages the enormous task of storing so much of our life in a readily accessible fashion involves the idea that experiences, as well as the neural mechanisms by which experiences are coded and recorded, are multidimensional. With this theoretical foreshadowing, let us consider observations made by Gail Risse on nonaphasic patients with left-hemisphere pathology who have to undergo cerebral angiography [19,23]. This is the medical procedure of injecting radio-paque dye into the carotid artery on either the left or the right side of the neck. This procedure is used to render the left or the right arterial system supplying the brain opaque to X-ray photography. It helps the neurologist and the neurosurgeon locate areas of brain damage due to tumors and other maladies.

When patients have to undergo angiography, the physician sometimes runs what is called an *amytal test* [24]. When the stopcock is switched at the point of injection, an anesthetic (sodium amytal) can be administered to one half of the brain, putting it to sleep, while leaving the opposite half-brain awake. Traditional speech and language tests are then run, so as to assure the physician that these processes are localized in the half-brain where they are sup-posed to be. Sometimes they are not, and it could be disastrous for the patient if surgery was carried out.

The tests of interest here are these. Prior to injection of the anesthetic, an object—for instance, a pencil—is placed in the left hand and out of view. The patient is asked to identify it. A correct identification signifies that the stereognostic, or touch, information has coursed normally from the left hand to the right hemisphere, where it is relayed via the corpus callosum to the speech mecha-nisms of the left hemisphere.

The left hemisphere is put to sleep, which means that the pa-tient is no longer conversant or capable of comprehending or pro-ducing natural language in any way. The opposite, right half of the body becomes flaccid. At the same time, however, the left half-body and the right hemisphere are both functional, because the drug affects only the injected side of the brain. Another object is placed in the left hand at this time, say, a spoon. The subject feels it, and after a few seconds, the spoon is removed. A few minutes later, the subject awakes, the drug having now dissipated, and the left hemisphere returns to consciousness.

The patient is asked, "What was placed in your hand?" and the typical response is, "Nothing," or, "I don't know." To test for a given recall ability, the patient is then asked, "What was placed in your hand before?" and he commonly says, "Do you mean the pencil?"

Even with the greatest amount of encouragement or prodding, no verbal report is forthcoming for the object placed in the hand during the anesthesia. A card with several objects attached to it is then placed in front of the patient, and almost immediately the left hand points to the object, in this case, the spoon.

One interpretation of this response is that information stored in the absence of language cannot be accessed by language when the verbal system reappears and becomes functional. The engram or memory for the spoon is encoded in neural language X, and speech is represented in neural language Y. The two languages are thus insulated from one another and are not conversant with each other inside the brain.

The model we are proposing here is that the normal brain is split into many domains. What can be done surgically and with sodium amytal are only exaggerated instances of a more general phenomenon, one that may prove to be a key to a viable model of mind. Pursuing this model, we turn to a corollary of the idea that information is multiply encoded, namely, that various aspects of experience are stored in multiple loci in the brain.

Multidimensionality of Experience and Information Storage

Our experiences are indeed multifaceted, and it is our view that different aspects of experience are differentially stored in the brain. Consider a recent clinical case that had a truly dramatic course.

The patient was a 62-year-old male surgeon with no known neurological disorders prior to a transitory stroke. He was a right-handed with left-hemisphere dominance for speech and language. He was intelligent, curious, and extremely positive about every aspect of the human condition. Accordingly, through all stages of the stroke, he was making every effort, using every faculty available to him, in trying to engage the environment.

On a Thursday evening following dinner, the patient complained of an excruciating headache followed by dizziness and vomiting. The following morning, he was taken to the hospital, where it was immediately diagnosed that a stroke had occurred. During the subsequent 72 hours, his speech and language facilities were disturbed, but there were no gross signs of paralysis or somatic sensory loss. There was a right homonymous hemianopsia. On Sunday morning his condition had deteriorated considerably and edema had set in. Steroids were administered and maintained for 48 hours. On the following Monday, the situation looked better, and during the following two weeks, a truly remarkable recovery occurred. Thus, within a 14-day period, a patient went from normal cognitive functioning into a state that totally disrupted these processes and back again to normal functioning. The observations to be reported here have to do with the course of recovery commencing 5 days after the onset of the stroke. It is the reconstruction of his cognitive and memory mechanisms that is of interest.

The main observations suggest that memory or engrams for things or events are multiply represented in the brain because the experiences themselves have multiple aspects. Thus, for example, when a red carnation was held up in full view and the patient was asked what it was, he said, "Flower." When asked what color, he said, "Red." But when the patient was asked what kind of flower, he was unable to say, "Carnation." Indeed, even when a list of names of familiar flowers was read aloud, he was still unable to make the match. This was true despite the fact that the patient's most active hobby was gardening. When the examiner finally said it was a carnation, the patient said the word aloud and accepted the carnation with equanimity. Then, spontaneously, the patient reached for the carnation, put it in his lapel, and smiled his satisfaction. At the same time in the recovery period, the patient asked about some flowers he and his daughter had planted "down by the road at the bottom of the hill." "What was that?" he asked. When the answer was given as gazania, a plant commonly known to him normally, he said, "Oh, gazania." Again, it seems that the category of names given to plants or flowers was not yet available for recall or recognition.

On the following day, when the edema had subsided even

more, thus making active more extensive brain areas, the patient was able to name all the flowers in the room (there was quite an assortment) with little or no difficulty.

These observations suggest that memory is multiply represented in the brain. The point is not that a particular engram associated with a particular experience is multiply represented but that a particular experience has multiple aspects to it and that these are stored at a variety of sites in the cerebrum. The prediction from such a model would be that when recall of an experience takes place in the presence of new brain damage, there may be a breakdown in the recalling of all aspects of the experience. In the present case, because of the transitory "turning off," as it were, of local neural processes, specific aspects of the past experience were not available to the subject. Clearly, normal experience has a "what" and "where" aspect. In the flower case above, the patient could remember "where" on the lot a plant had been planted but could not remember "what" until the part of the brain that had stored the "what" information had returned to normal functioning.

Of course, this kind of analysis is less fashionable today than those models favoring a more general loss of memory function. Yet, one must keep in mind the variety of diseases that produce disturbances in memory function. Also, unless the patient's personal history is extremely well known to the examiner, the probability of uncovering a lacuna is low. Analysis of the memory function of an unfamiliar patient finds one on a fishing expedition, trying to find a subject area in which a specific loss might be detected. Yet, with a little practice, one becomes fairly adept at zeroing in on the appropriate subject matter.

Clinical observations of this nature lead us to speculate that in normal man there may well exist a variety of separate memory banks, each inherently coherent, organized, and logical and with its own set of values. These memory banks do not necessarily communicate with one another inside the brain. If this is true, then the only way for the organism—which is to say, the cognitive subsystem in the forefront of consciousness at any one point in time, which is the verbal system in humans—to discover its total resources is to watch itself as it behaves. If memory bank A takes control of the motor apparatus and produces a behavior, it is only subsequent to the event that the other memory systems become aware that such impulses, so to speak, have been stored in the brain. This idea foreshadows our view of some mechanisms of consciousness in the next chapter.

In this regard, it is worth noting the considerable mass of psychological data revealing that within a given class or "memory network," there are distinct differences in retrieval time for the "calling up" of related elements[20]. This time difference suggests that such information may be located in spatially separate points in the brain.

Thus, we feel that there are good reasons for believing that there is no unitary mechanism responsible for the encoding of information in the brain and that all the information in the brain is not mutually accessible. If this is true, of course, the task of the neuroscientist is slightly more complex than has been supposed, if that is possible. We may be faced with the fact that memory storage, encoding, and decoding is a multifaceted process that is multiply represented in the brain.

Implications for a Theory of Memory

It is interesting to examine some of the traditional views on memory mechanisms as viewed in this new light. Many, in fact, are consistent with this model. The new idea again is that the normal brain has a variety of coherent and viable information-storage systems, each largely independent and isolated from the other.

The memory mechanism that psychologists have been studying ad nauseum is the verbal processing system. Yet, what if this is but one of the systems of memory and, while it is working away, simultaneous activity is going on in several other nonverbal systems, which have gestures and movements as their own modes of response? In other words, what if the memory systems that exist—say, in nonspeaking animals—are also present and working in us along with our admittedly unique language and speech systems? If such an arrangement exists in man, then one can indeed look at an embarrassingly huge number of previous studies on human memory and come to some unique conclusions about their meaning.

The classic distinction, for example, between recognition and recall dissolves almost immediately. This distinction, of course, is the well-reported and widely experienced phenomenon that a person can recall only a small part of a body of information given to him, whereas he can recognize a great deal more. In the present model, the recall phase is only calling upon the verbal system for response. The verbal system, however, reports only a small amount of information because as with the other independent systems, it has a limited capacity. When the recognition phase is introduced, however, the name of the game becomes quite different. Now, the nonverbal systems have an opportunity to express themselves by pointing to a series of objects, and with that response possible, all the information that the multiple nonverbal systems have stored can be reported, making the entire system appear more resourceful.

Recognition tests have long been considered to be more of a sensitive measure for information stored because they allow for expression of stimuli stored with weaker values of some kind or another. In the present model, such a continuum between recognition and recall skills becomes more the product of the expression of several equally capable storage systems, each given an equal chance to demonstrate what it knows.

There is another aspect to this model. Psychologists have for years been trying to understand the network of our associative memory. The assumption is that it is huge and complex and is interrelated in some kind of mind-boggling way. What is being argued here would encourage quite a different model. While associations surely exist, the degree of interconnection need not be so extensive. The verbal system, while having nonverbal associations, could also become aware of knowledge possessed by one of the nonverbal systems by observing emitted behavior, which is to say, stored information.

One can find experimental data from a variety of quarters that complement this proposal. For example, in dichotic listening studies, it has been widely observed that information is normally suppressed and not subsequently recognized from one ear when a subject is asked to actively process information presented to the other ear. This is true, however, only when the secondary information is of the same kind being processed by the subject's first ear. If the information is different, thereby possibly allowing a different memory bank to be used, it is found that the information is stored and is later available, as revealed by subsequent recognition tests.

It is interesting to reexamine the literature on the tonic effect that cuing has on assisting recall in this light. When a past experience is to be remembered, it is prima facie a multidimensional experience involving time, space, colors, sounds, smell, temperature, and a variety of other stimuli. Many of these are not activated when one is called upon to relate an old memory verbally, and as a result, the verbal memory is limited in extent. When a person reenters the physical circumstance of the memory, however, the ability to recall verbal aspects of the event is usually increased. Clearly, a facilitory effect of having the dormant system activated by being in the physical surroundings has a tonic effect on the verbal recall.

If one proviso is added to the model being suggested, then the opportunity for explaining memory data becomes almost limitless. It is a safety feature primarily and consists of the fact that when information of a perceptual nature, regardless of the input modality, is encoded with language systems active, the information is encoded verbally as well as nonverbally, and a bond or association is formed that allows the language system some access to these stored memories laid down by nonverbal systems. Since in the adult it is the usual state of affairs to have the language system free to develop such bonds and thereby free access to information stored in the nonverbal systems, the model we are proposing here would never occur to one considering the standard experimental results. It would only fall out of neuroclinical observation, which is to say, in passing, that studying the abnormal case is a rich way of understanding normal processes.

REFERENCES

1. D. Hume, 1949, first published in 1739, *A Treatise on Human Nature*, Oxford, Clarendon Press.
2. L. R. Brooks, 1968, Spatial and verbal components of the act of recall, *Can. J. Psychol. 22:*349–368.
3. S. J. Segal, 1971, *Imagery*, New York, Academic Press.
4. U. Neisser, 1967, *Cognitive Psychology*, New York, Appleton Press.
5. P. W. Sheehan, 1966, Functional similarity of imaging to perceiving, *Percept. Mot. Skills,* monograph supplement, *6-V23:*1011–1033.
6. S. J. Segal and P. Gordon, 1969, The Perky effect revisited, *Percept. Mot. Skills 28:*791–797.
7. S. J. Segal and V. Fusella, 1970, Influence of imagined pictures and sounds on detection of auditory and visual signals, *J. Exp. Psychol. 83:*458–464.
8. J. D. Johnson and M. S. Gazzaniga, 1970, Interhemisphere imitation in split-brain monkeys, *Exp. Neurol. 27:*206–212.
9. J. D. Johnson and M. S. Gazzaniga, 1971, Some effects of non-reinforcement in split-brain monkeys, *Exp. Neurol. 33:*412–419.
10. C. Trevarthen, 1962, Double visual learning in split-brain monkeys, *Science 136:*258.
11. M. S. Gazzaniga, 1973, Discrimination learning without reward, *Physiol. Behav. 11:*121–123.
12. C. L. Hull, 1952, *A Behavior System,* New Haven, Conn., Yale University Press.
13. R. Nakamura and M. S. Gazzaniga, 1975, Interhemispheric relations in split-brain monkeys, *Fed. Proc. 32:*367a.
14. A. R. Gibson and M. S. Gazzaniga, 1971, Differences in eating behavior in split-brain monkeys, *Physiologist 50:*14.
15. A. R. Gibson, 1972, Independence of cortico-hypothalamic mechanisms in brain-bisected monkeys, unpublished doctoral thesis, NYU, New York.
16. D. Premack, 1965, Reinforcement theory, in: *Nebraska Symposium on Motivation 13:*129–148, Lincoln, Neb., University of Nebraska Press.
17. B. F. Skinner, 1953, *Science and Human Behavior,* New York, Macmillan Press.
18. M. S. Gazzaniga, I. S. Szer, and A. M. Crane, 1974, Modification of drinking behavior in the adipsic rat, *Exp. Neurol. 42:*483–489.
19. G. L. Risse and M. S. Gazzaniga, 1976, Verbal retrieval of right hemisphere memories established in the absence of language, *Neurology 26:*354.
20. A. Collins and R. Quillian, 1969, Retrieval time from semantic memory, *J. Verb. Learn. Verb. Behav. 8:*240.
21. M. S. Gazzaniga, 1976, The biology of memory, in: M. Rosenweig and M. Bennet (Eds.), *Neuroscience: A Review,* Cambridge, Mass., MIT Press.
22. G. Risse, J. E. LeDoux, and M. S. Gazzaniga, unpublished observations.

23. M. S. Gazzaniga, 1972, One brain—two minds? *Am. Sci. 60:*311–317.

24. J. A. Wada and T. Rasmussen, 1962, Intracarotid injection of sodium amytal for the lateralization of cerebral dominance: Experimental and clinical observations, *J. Neurosurg. 17:*266–282.

25. N. Geschwind, 1965, Disconnexion syndrome in animals and man, *Brain 88:*237–294, 564–585.

26. D. O. Hebb, 1968, On imagery, *Psychol. Rev. 75:*466–477.

On the Mechanisms
of Mind

When the inevitable topic of consciousness is approached in the light of modern brain research, the experienced student has come to brace himself for the mellifluous intonations of someone's personal experience and ideas on the matter, as opposed to data. Yet, we all listen dutifully, because ultimately the business of the serious neuroscientist is to figure out the mechanisms of brain and mind.

One of the most thoughtful and experienced neuroscientists in the world on this issue is Roger W. Sperry. According to Sperry, consciousness is an "emergent property of cerebral activity . . . and is an integral component of the brain process that functions as an essential constituent action, and exerts a directive wholistic form of control over the flow pattern of cerebral excitation"[1].

Thus, Sperry, after years of thought, feels it necessary to instruct a beleaguered yet lackadaisical field of professional brain and behavior scientists that mental properties of the brain are real and that they can exert control over the individual neural elements that upon interaction give rise to mental phenomena. It is testimony to the thinking at the time on the subject that this needed saying, and Sperry's papers, as usual, are extremely important in focusing future work on important questions. Yet, in no way should such overviews be construed as insights into the mechanism of consciousness per se. These types of analyses deal with consciousness as a single impenetrable entity.

The operational properties and mechanisms of conscious experience thus remain largely unidentified. Yet, it is to this area that we personally find our own research program directed, and it is our experimental studies on the "how" of consciousness that occupy this chapter.

We will describe our observations on one truly exceptional individual, case P.S. P.S.'s uniqueness amongst split-brain patients centers around the psychological robustness of his right hemisphere. As described in Chapter 4, although only his left hemisphere can talk, other linguistic skills are extensively represented in both half-brains, and most of what follows deals with observations made possible by this special neurological circumstance.

SPLIT CONSCIOUSNESS

Much of the intrique surrounding the split-brain studies of the early 1960s was related to the possibility that the mechanisms of human consciousness were doubly represented following brain bisection. While the conscious properties of the left hemisphere were apparent through the patients' verbal behavior, the view that the right hemisphere was also worthy of conscious status was widely criticized. Sir John Eccles, for example, asserted that the psychological capacities of the right hemisphere were best described as "automatisms"[2]. Others, such as Donald MacKay, argued that unless it could be shown that each separated half-brain has its own independent system for subjectively assigning values to events and setting goals and reponse priorities, the split brain could not be viewed as a split mind[3].

In a series of tests aimed at specifying the nature and extent of linguistic rpresentation in P.S.'s right hemisphere, we lateralized pictures of objects to his mute half-brain and asked him to spell the name of the object by selecting letters from a group and arranging them in proper sequence (see Chapter 4). His capacity to respond in this situation raised the question of whether he might also be able to spell his answer to subjective and personal questions directed to his mute hemisphere. This seemed to be the opportunity to assess whether the right hemisphere, along with the left, could possess conscious properties following brain bisection.

We generated a series of questions that could be visually presented exclusively to the right hemisphere[4]. This was accomplished by verbally stating the question, except that key words in the question were replaced by the word blank and then the missing information was exposed in the left-visual field, which effectively lateralized visual input to the right half-brain. Subsequently, P.S. was asked to spell his answer by selecting and arranging letters from two complete alphabets (made up of Scrabble letters).

The first question asked was "Who *blank*?" The key words lateralized to the right hemisphere on this trial were *are you*. Our expectations were met! As his eyes scanned the 52 letters available, his left hand reached out and selected the *P*, set it down, and then proceeded to collect the remaining letters needed to spell *Paul* (Figure 40). Overflowing with excitement, having just communicated on a personal level with a right hemisphere, we collected ourselves, and then initiated the next trial by saying, "Would you spell your favorite *blank*?" Then *girl* appeared in the left visual field. Out came the left hand again, and this time it spelled *Liz*, the name of his girlfriend at the time. On the next two trials, the question was the same, but the key words were *person* and then *hobby*. *Car* was the reply to hobby, and *Heney Wi Fozi* was the response to his favorite person. (Henry Winkler is the real-life name of the television character Fonzie, whom P.S., a fifteen year old boy, idolizes). Another question was, "What is tomorrow?" He correctly spelled *Sunday*. He spelled *automobile race* as the job he would pick. This is most interesting, because the left hemisphere frequently asserts that he wants to be a draftsman. In fact, shortly after the test session, we asked P.S. what sort of job he would like to have, and the left hemisphere said, "Oh, be a draftsman." Finally, we asked the right hemisphere to spell its "mood." It spelled *good*.

These observations suggested to us that the right hemisphere in P.S. possesses qualities that are deserving of conscious status. His right hemisphere has a sense of self, for it knows the name it

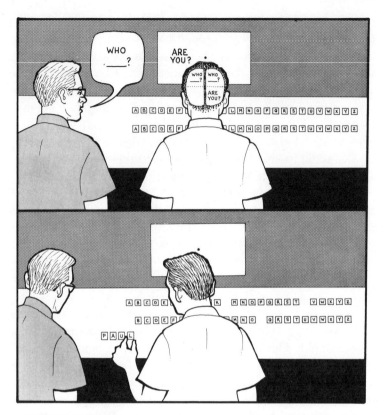

FIGURE 40. Volitional expression by the mute hemisphere (see text).

collectively shares with the left. It has feelings, for it can describe its mood. It has a sense of who it likes and what it likes, for it can name its favorite people and its favorite hobby. The right hemisphere in P.S. also has a sense of the future, for it knows what day tomorrow is. Furthermore, it has goals and aspirations for the future, for it can name its occupational choice.

It is important to emphasize that these responses were self-generated by P.S.'s right hemisphere from a set of infinite possibilities. The only aid provided was the two alphabets, from which he could select letters at will. The fact that this mute half-brain could generate personal answers to ambiguous and subjective questions demonstrates that in P.S., the right hemisphere has its own independent response-priority–determining mechanisms, which is to say, its own volitional control system.

Thus, it would appear that the right hemisphere, along with but independent of the left, *can* possess conscious properties following brain bisection. In other words, the mechanisms of human consciousness *can* be split and doubled by split-brain surgery.

Because P.S. is the first split-brain patient to clearly possess double consciousness, it seems that if we could identify the factor that distinguishes his right hemisphere from the right hemisphere of other split-brain patients, we would have a major clue to the underlying nature of conscious processes. That factor is undoubtedly the extensive linguistic representation in P.S.'s right hemisphere. As we have seen, his right hemisphere can spell, and in addition, it can comprehend verbal commands, as well as process other parts of speech and make conceptual judgments involving verbal information. While it is possible that the conscious properties observed in his right hemisphere are spuriously associated with these linguistic skills, the fact remains that in all other patients, where linguistic sophistication is lacking in the right hemisphere, so too is the evidence for consciousness.

Observations such as these immediately raise the question of whether nonhuman organisms are conscious. However, the clear distinction between the conscious status of the left and right hemispheres of most split-brain patients (P.S. excluded) adds an important qualification to this question. Unless it could be shown that nonhumans possess conscious powers that surpass those of the right hemisphere of most split-brain patients, then the criticisms (see earlier discussion) levied against the conscious status of these right hemispheres also apply to nonhumans. Still, it is not our intent to deny the possibility of some form of conscious awareness in nonhumans. Instead, our point is that while nonhumans may be found to be aware and even self-aware, they are nevertheless not aware in the unique ways and to the extent made possible by the human verbal system. Consequently, our aim in the following is to identify and examine some of the mechanisms through which the verbal system contributes to consciousness, as we as humans experience it.

VERBAL ATTRIBUTION AND THE SOCIOLOGY OF MIND

The person is engaged in much more activity than can possibly enter consciousness at once, and in our opinion, much of what does enter is what is registered by the verbal system. It is the one system that is capable of continuously monitoring our overt behavioral activities, as well as our perceptions, thoughts, and moods. In taking note of, integrating, and interpreting these events, we believe that the verbal system provides for a personal sense of conscious reality.

In the following, we will examine how further observations on case P.S. shed light on these mechanisms. Again, it is only through the novel experimental situation involved in testing such a patient that these mechanisms, which we feel are basic to man, are exposed.

As a result of having bilateral representation of language comprehension, P.S. is able to act in response to verbal commands exclusively presented to either hemisphere but can describe verbally only the left-hemisphere stimuli. The observations of relevance here involve the manner in which his left hemisphere dealt with our queries as to why he was responding in a certain way to commands known directly by the right half-brain alone. In brief, when P.S. was asked, "Why are you doing that?" his talking left hemisphere was faced with the cognitive problem of explaining a discrete overt movement of great clarity carried out for reasons truly unknown to it.

The left hemisphere proved extremely adept at immediately attributing cause to the action. When *laugh,* for example, was presented to the right hemisphere, the subject commenced laughing and, when asked why, said, "Oh, you guys are really something" (Figure 41). When the command *rub* was flashed, the subject, with the left hand, rubbed the back of his head. When asked what the command was, he said "Itch." Here again, the response was observed by the left hemisphere, and the subject immediately characterized it. Yet that he said "itch" instead of "rub" shows that he was guessing. In the same way, he could be quite accurate when the command had less leeway for mul-

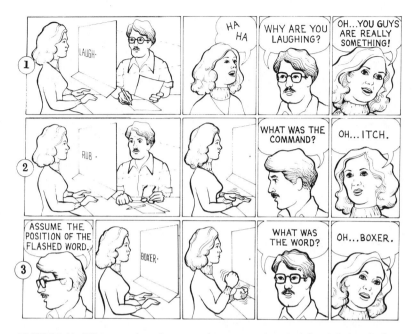

FIGURE 41. When a series of commands were presented to the right hemisphere, each evoked a response. Although the left hemisphere did not know what the command was, it attempted to account for the response. When the command was *laugh* or *rub,* the left hemisphere instantly "filled in." When the response was less equivocal, the reason generated for the action was quite accurate, as with the word *boxer.*

tiple description, as in the case of the word *boxer.* The test instruction was to "assume the position of. . . ." The subject correctly assumed the pugilistic position, and when asked what the word was, he said, "Boxer." But on subsequent trials, when he was restrained and the word *boxer* was flashed, the left hemisphere said it saw nothing. Moments later, when released, however, he assumed the position, and said, "O.K., it was *boxer.*"

Similar responses were observed in other tests. Pictures of objects were lateralized to his right hemisphere and P.S. was required to spell out the name of the object by selecting and arranging Scrabble letters, as described earlier. If while spelling the word he was asked to name the object he had seen, the left hemisphere's verbal response was consistent with the information available, but inconsistent with the true state of affairs known only by the right hemisphere. For example, after the picture of a playing card was flashed to his right hemisphere and he began to select the letters, we asked P.S. what the object was. Looking down at the letters *c a r,* he said "car." However, as this response was being emitted by the left hemisphere, the left hand and the right hemisphere completed the word by adding the final letter *d*. The left hemisphere then said, "Oh, it was a card," and P.S. smiled.

In another series of observations, we simultaneously presented each hemisphere with a different object–picture, and the subject was required to select the picture choice cards that best related to the flashed stimuli. Thus, if a "cherry" was one of the stimuli flashed, the correct answer might have been "apple," as opposed to "toaster," "chicken," or "glass," with the superordinate concept being, of course, "fruit." Using this procedure (which was developed by Marjorie Pinsley for testing aphasic patients) we found it possible to escalate the subtlety of the cognitive requirement without changing the test design or the response demands upon the subject.

It was clear that each hemisphere under the simultaneous presentation could perform. Only rarely did the response of one side block a response from the other. In general, each hemisphere pointed to the correct answer on each trial.

What is of particular interest, however, is the way the subject verbally interpreted these double-field responses. When a snow scene was presented to the right hemisphere and a chicken claw was presented to the left, P.S. quickly and dutifully responded correctly by choosing a picture of a chicken from a series of four cards with his right hand and a picture of a shovel from a series of four cards with his left hand. The subject was then asked, "What did you see?" "I saw a claw and I picked the chicken, and you have to clean out the chicken shed with a shovel" (Figure 42).

In trial after trial, we saw this kind of response. The left hemisphere could easily and accurately identify why it had picked the answer, and then subsequently, and without batting an eye, it

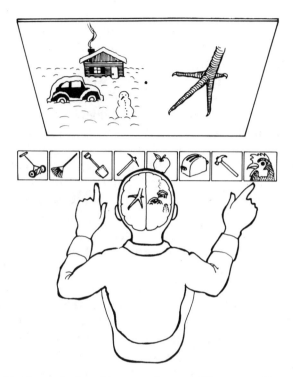

FIGURE 42. The method used in presenting two different cognitive tasks simultaneously, one to each hemisphere. The left hemisphere was required to process the answer to the chicken claw, while the right dealt with the implications of being presented with a snow scene. After each hemisphere responded, the left hemisphere was asked to explain its choices. See text for implications.

would incorporate the right hemisphere's response into the framework. While we knew exactly why the right hemisphere had made its choice, the left hemisphere could merely guess. Yet, the left did not offer its suggestion in a guessing vein but rather as a statement of fact as to why that card had been picked.

These varied observations on P.S. offer us the opportunity to consider whether we were not observing a basic mental mechanism common to us all. We feel that the conscious verbal self is not always privy to the origin of our actions, and when it observes the person behaving for unknown reasons, it attributes cause to the action as if it knows but in fact it does not. It is as if the verbal self looks out and sees whăt the person is doing, and from that knowledge it interprets a reality. This notion is reminiscent of the well-known theory of cognitive dissonance, which suggests how one's sense of reality, one's system of beliefs about the world, arises as a consequence of considering what one does[5].

Implicit in the idea that self-consciousness involves, at least in part, verbal consideration of sensorimotor activities is the assumption that the person or self is not a unified psychological entity, so that the conscious verbal self comes to know the other selves through overt behavior. In other words, what we are again (see Chapter 6) suggesting is that there are multiple mental systems in the brain, each with the capacity to produce behavior, and each with its own impulses for action, and these systems are not necessarily conversant internally. This point was well illustrated by the results of the sodium amytal experiment[6] described in the previous chapter. In brief, the data suggested that information encoded while the left hemisphere was anesthetized was uninterpretable by the verbal system when the left hemisphere returned to normal functioning. In other words, the verbal system seems to encode information in its special way, and the other mental systems do the same. So when information is encoded by other than the verbal system, the person is not consciously aware of the information.

These observations allow for a rather radical hypothesis. Could it be that in the developing organism a constellation of mental systems (emotional, motivational, perceptual, and so on) exists, each with its own values and response probabilities? Then, as maturation continues, the behaviors that these separate systems emit are monitored by the one system we come to use more and more, namely, the verbal, natural language system. Gradually, a concept of self-control develops so that the verbal self comes to know the impulses for action that arise from the other selves, and it either tries to inhibit these impulses or free them, as the case may be.

The model being proposed here, then, is clear. We believe that the split-brain observations, combined with the sodium amytal data, paint a unique view of the mental properties of the brain. The mind is not a psychological entity but a sociological entity, being composed of many submental systems. What can be done surgically and through hemisphere anesthetization are only exaggerated instances of a more general phenomenon. The uniqueness of man, in this regard, is his ability to verbalize and, in so doing, create a personal sense of conscious reality out of the multiple mental systems present.

EMOTION AND CONSCIOUSNESS

The next set of observations to be described here provide new insights into the nature of cognitive-emotional interactions and, at the same time, point out how the verbal system is capable of monitoring internal psychological states in addition to overt behavioral activities.

On the verbal commands test described earlier, where a word was lateralized to the right hemisphere and P.S. was instructed to perform the action described by the word, his reaction to the word *kiss* proved revealing[7]. Although the left hemisphere of this adolescent boy did not see the word, immediately after *kiss* was exposed to the mute right hemisphere, the left blurted out, "Hey, no way, no way. You've got to be kidding." When asked what it was that he was not going to do, he was unable to tell us. Later, we presented *kiss* to the left hemisphere and a similar response occurred: "No way. I'm not going to kiss you guys." However, this time the speaking half-brain knew what the word was. In both instances, the command *kiss* elicited an emotional reaction that was detected by the verbal system of the left hemisphere, and the overt verbal response of the left hemisphere was basically the same, regardless of whether the command was presented to the right or left half-brain. In other words, the verbal system of the left hemisphere seemed to be able to accurately read the emotional tone and direction of a word seen by the right hemisphere alone.

This observation, which suggests that emotion is neurally encoded in a directionally specific manner, is inconsistent with the currently accepted cognitive theory of emotion[8]. According to the cognitive theory, the neural and other physiological mechanisms underlying emotional experience only provide a nonspecific state of arousal, with the direction of arousal being determined by the cognitive apprehension of the external situation in which the arousal occurs. However, in P.S., the left hemisphere appeared to have experienced a directionally specific emotion in the absence of a cognition. The following experiment was thus aimed at evaluating the reality of this phenomenon.

We selected a number of words that repeatedly appear in P.S.'s verbal behavior. It was assumed that personal words would be more likely to elicit measurable emotional responses than neutral words. Following the lateralized visual exposure of a word, P.S. was encouraged to verbally rate the word on a preference scale. The scale values included "like very much," "like," "undecided," "dislike," and "dislike very much." When the word was presented to the left hemisphere, the verbal judgment was made by the hemisphere that saw the word. However, when the word was lateralized to the right hemisphere, the left hemisphere had to verbally respond to a word it did not see.

We obtained 21 left-hemisphere ratings of words lateralized to the right hemisphere. There were 12 right-hemisphere words rated, some as many as 3 times, others only once.

Figure 43 compares the left-hemisphere rating of each word on the first left-hemisphere trial with the first successful right-hemisphere trial (an unsuccessful right-hemisphere trial was one on which the word could be named; such ratings were counted as left-hemisphere trials). In only one instance ("Nixon") did the left-hemisphere rating of right-hemisphere words differ by more than one scale value from the left-hemisphere rating of the same words after left-hemisphere exposure.

It thus appears that the emotional value of a stimulus can be neurally encoded in a directionally specific manner. Although the perceptual nature of stimuli exposed to the right hemisphere was unavailable to the left hemisphere, the emotional value of the stimuli was nevertheless available to the left hemisphere. Such observations suggest to us that while cognitions can surely initiate emotional responses, and while the visceral (sympathetic) arousal in

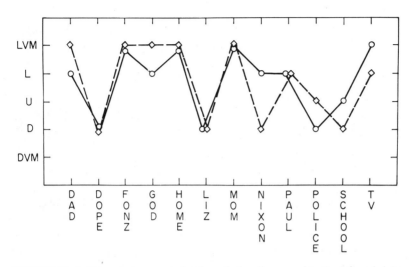

FIGURE 43. Left hemisphere verbal rating of stimuli exposed to the left and right hemispheres. Data points represented by open squares connected by dotted lines indicate right hemisphere exposure, and open circles connected by solid lines indicate left hemisphere exposure. In only one instance ("Nixon") did the ratings differ by more than one scale value.

emotion is nonspecific, the brain does indeed play an important role in determining the nature of experienced emotions. While this point is all too obvious, its implications have been overshadowed by the "black-box" view of emotional mechanisms that has resulted from a straightforward acceptance of the cognitive theory.

What possible mechanisms could be involved in the type of emotional encoding suggested here? As noted, P.S. is a callosum-sectioned patient, which means his anterior commissure was surgically spared. Anatomical studies have shown that the human anterior commissure derives its fibers from the temporal lobe and from subcortical "limbic" structures, in particular, the amygdala, and projects to the same regions in the other hemisphere[9]. Evidence that the interhemispheric limbic connections are intact and functioning in P.S. is provided by our observation that like other anterior commissure-intact patients and unlike split-brain patients with anterior commissure sections, P.S. shows interhemispheric transfer of olfactory information (see Chapter 2). Given the presumed role of limbic structures in emotion, in addition to olfaction, the interlimbic connections of the anterior commissure could well be responsible for the interhemispheric emotional judgments observed in P.S.

It is important to distinguish these observations on P.S. from previous observations on patients whose surgeries included the anterior commissure in addition to the corpus callosum. In particular, on one occasion case N.G., upon being presented with a picture of a nude woman in the left visual field, giggled. When asked why she was laughing, she responded, "That's a funny machine." This is more appropriately interpreted as an instance of attributing cause to behavior of unknown origin than as an instance of emotional transfer, for the left hemisphere judgment ("That's a funny machine") was based on an externally observable action (laughter).

At the psychological level, the observation that the verbal system can accurately read the emotional tone precipitated by an external stimulus without knowing the nature of the stimulus allows speculation concerning the nature and variability of our mood states. In brief, the idea that we are intrigued with is that a person is not always aware of the origin of his moods, just as he or she is not always aware of the origin of his or her actions. In other words, the conscious self appears to be capable of noticing that the person is in a particular mood without knowing why. It is as if we can become subtly conditioned to particular visual, somatosensory, auditory, olfactory, and gustatory stimuli. While such conditioning can be within the realm of awareness of the conscious self, it is not necessarily so. When in Florence, for example, one can be focused on David and feel so aroused, awed, and inspired that unknown to the verbal system the brain is also recording the scents, noises and the total Gestalt of that most remarkable city. The emotional tone conditioned to these subtle aspects of the experience might later be triggered in other settings because of the presence of similar or related stimuli. This person, puzzled by his affective state, might ask himself, "Why do I feel so good today?" At this point if the Florentine experience is not recalled (registered by the verbal system), the process of verbal attribution might take over and concoct a substitute, though perhaps very plausible, explanation. In short, the environment has ways of planting hooks in our minds, and while the verbal system may not know the why or what of it all, part of its job is to make sense out of the emotional and other mental systems and, in so doing, allow man, with his mental complexity, the illusion of a unified self.

We thus feel that the verbal system's role in creating our sense of conscious reality is crucial and enormous. It is the system that is continually observing our actual behavior as well as our cognitions and internal moods. In attributing cause to behavioral and psychological states, an attitudinal view of the world involving beliefs and values is constructed, and this view becomes a dominant theme in our own self-image.

Given this overview, it is instructional to consider some of the major issues of psychology and philosophy and to see how they fit into this neurologically based model. We begin with an example of cognitive dissonance and then consider the problem of free will.

WHY THE NEED FOR CONSONANCE?

One of the more powerful ideas on the nature of behavioral processes ever stated was the theory of cognitive dissonance[5]. In broad terms, the phenomenon is this: when a person's beliefs, opinions, or attitudes are met with disagreement as a consequence of a freely produced behavior of his own, a state of dissonance obtains. His cognition prior to his behavior is in conflict with his just-completed behavior, and that state of dissonance is not allowed by the organism. Consonance is demanded and is usually achieved by a change in the prior value or belief.

Let's take an imaginary example. George is married and full of fidelity. Then a set of circumstances develops that finds George involved in an affair with another woman. George does not believe in such behavior and does not condone extramarital affairs. So, immediately after the experience, George is very much in a state of dissonance concerning his recent behavior. George initially attributes it to being drunk or being seduced. That helps, but George is soon in bed again with his new friend. As the affair continues, his dissonance increases and something must change. What usually changes is George's attitude about his marriage. Before long, he attributes his behavior to domestic tensions and comes to believe they are much worse than he had previously thought. As a result, George shortly finds himself in divorce court. He has concluded that he must be having the affair because his marriage was foul. These rationalizations and actions are the changes that resolve George's dissonance. Divorce becomes an unavoidable consequence. George's fate was sealed, in a sense, after the first night.

George could have achieved consonance by changing other values. He divorced because he clung to the idea that married people are, among other things, supposed to be faithful. If George had changed his ideas on fidelity in marriage, he could have achieved consonance.

There are millions of examples of dissonance theory at work, and hundreds have been worked out under strict experimental conditions in the laboratory. What is not understood is why the organism seeks consonance. Why can't dissonance be a viable and chronic state for the biological organism?

Let's take a step back and consider a prior question. Why did George suddenly find himself in bed with Molly in the first place? What is the mechanism for eliciting a dissonant behavior from the beginning? The behavior was clearly contrary to his existing (verbally stored) belief about such matters, and normally the verbal system can exert self-control. The reason we propose is that yet another information system with a different reference and a different set of values existed in George, but because it was encoded in a particular way, its existence was not known to George's verbal system and therefore was outside of its control. This other system wasn't known to the dominant verbal system until the day it grabbed hold and elicited a behavioral act that caused great consternation to his verbal system. This other side of George was not known to him until a set of environmental and biological circumstances came together and elicited this new behavior. Once elicited, however, George's verbal system had no choice but to account for it and to adjust his verbal perceptions and guidelines for behavior in such a way as to take this newly discovered aspect of his personality into account. In this view, it is the verbal system that is the final arbiter of our multiple mental systems, many of which we come to know only by actually behaving. Emitted and elicited behaviors are important ways of discovering the multiple selves dwelling inside. Behavior is a key way that these separate information systems can communicate with each other. As we noted in the last chapter, such mechanisms greatly reduce the extent of internal association networks that would otherwise have to be postulated to explain memory capacity.

Cross-Cuing

Let us go back a moment and cite some work with split-brain monkeys that dramatically reveals these same kinds of phenomena. Clearly, in the split-brain case, in which there is an actual surgical intervention to produce, at a minimum, a double mental system, the phenomenon of one mental system's watching another and, as a result, altering its behavior is explicitly present. As with the amytal study, it seems to illustrate possible normal mechanisms.

In the split-brain monkey, the information necessary to solve a visual problem can be divided up so that some aspects of the problem go to one hemisphere and some go to the other. It has been maintained that such problems can be solved, at least in part, with some practice. It is unlikely that the information is integrated neurally, as it were. Instead, cross-cuing strategies seem to be involved in such instances[10-12]. A most elegant demonstration of this in animal work has come from Charles Hamilton's experiments on a matching-to-sample task in the monkey[13].

Hamilton presented the sample stimulus of a pattern discrimination to one hemisphere and the matching stimuli to the other. For example, the left brain might see a "plus." In order for the animal to perform the task, the right hemisphere must know whether the left saw a "plus" or a "zero," because, in this case, it would push the "plus" button for a peanut reward. A normal monkey with the brain unsplit can do this task instantly and with ease. What Hamilton discovered is that a split-brain monkey can do the same after some practice. This finding is reminiscent of earlier work by Colwyn Trevarthen, and in his hands, this outcome meant that there were subcortical exchange systems serving to integrate the split-visual information[14]. Hamilton, however, pursued the cross-cuing notion and made the prediction that if the right hemisphere was choosing correctly because of some *behavioral* cue produced by the left hemisphere, it ought not to make a difference what the stimulus was that the left saw. So instead of presenting to the left the well-trained plus or zero, he showed it a new stimulus. The right then saw this stimulus and another novel one. The animal didn't hesitate and immediately performed at a high level because the right was not responding to the visual cue per se but to flinch or a head bob or a grunt that the left hemisphere reliably made to one stimulus. We have, then, mental system right, looking at the behavior of mental system left, and through the behavioral cuing strategies, the two systems communicate.

Developmental Aspects

An enormous consideration for the reliability of this overall model for normal processes involves determining how separate neural storage systems would naturally develop in man. That is, since most of our experiences are ongoing at a time when our verbal system is alert, it would seem at first glance to be unlikely that information is stored in the verbal system's absence, thereby making the information inaccessible to language.

Yet, there is the critical period during development before language is a functional mechanism. During this period, important conditioning that bears fruit for a variety of adult motivational states is surely ongoing. Responses and attitudes of all kinds associated with interpersonal relations are extensively examined by the young child when considering the smile or the frown of those around him, and these play a huge role in controlling behavior. The behavioral tone of the emerging adult is largely set in these preverbal years, and adult impulses—which is to say, response patterns—can largely be determined by the early associations.

Years later, these early states can emerge, to the total surprise of the verbal system.

In the adult stage, the normally involved language system can be so busy and active that information bypasses its processes and becomes stored without the verbal system's noting it. An example here comes from the common experience of being able to find one's way home from a new place even though the verbal system was engaged (say, through conversation) during the entire experience with the new route. If called upon to state the way, the verbal system could not do it. Yet, once on the way, the critical roads are recognized, and the proper choices for direction are made.

THE MULTIPLE SELF AND FREE WILL

The last implication of this model that we would like to consider surfaces right on the question of the nature of personal responsibility. Most of our social institutions are built on the notion that man is personally responsible for his actions, and implicit in that statement is a notion that man has a unitary nature embodied in the self. What are we now to do with that view, given the possibility that multiple selves exist, each of which can control behavior at various moments in time?

Let us begin by examining the concept of free will as it has stood up in our scientific age. This examination is extremely important because the issue of responsibility (whether personal or social) is usually argued on the merits of a unitary self and the concept of free will. Up until recently, the scientific community had pretty much written off such ideas as free will, viewing them as holdovers from the Dark Ages. Science is reductionistic by nature, and many scientists believe in fact that the world is as mechanical as clockwork. Things don't just happen. There are inputs to every system, and knowing the inputs will find one able to explain and predict the outputs. That's the line of thought, at any rate.

At the level of human behavior, this means that when one feels that he or she is freely choosing which lad or lass to marry, he or she is, in fact, reacting in the only way possible to a set of forces working upon him or her. That the decision is made freely is a pure illusion. Behavior is the lawful and exacting product of past experience, according to behaviorists and reductionists.

Many people have tried to argue their way out of this rather depressing dilemma. The lively journalist Garry Wills examined the problem in his book on Catholicism with the notion that man gains more freedom by knowing more[15]. That kind of analysis, of course, misses the point, but it is one that reflects much of the thinking on the problem. Still others, who are more scientifically trained, have invoked Heisenberg's uncertainty principle, but that, upon careful analysis, proves to be inappropriate when one is considering basic neural phenomena.

One who has really addressed the issue is D. M. MacKay[16]. He has dealt with the problem head on and puts man right back on top and in personal control of behavior. The argument goes like this.

Man can be considered as mechanistic as clockwork and still be considered to be personally responsible for his actions. That is, he is personally free in his decisions. This is true because, put simply, if you tell someone that he will eat apples for lunch because of some fantastic knowledge you possess of his past behavior, all he has to do to prove you wrong is not to eat apples. At first glance, there would seem to be an easy solution. The next time, the person will not be told what the predictor predicts about his behavior. Instead, it will be written down, and after the critical event, the prediction will be examined, and with this condition, the predictor will prove to be correct.

That still won't work, however, as MacKay has pointed out, because, if one thinks carefully about it, in order for something to be true, it must be valid for all people. The critical point here is that while the prediction may be true for the predictor, it is not binding on our victim and consequently not valid for both parties. A true and valid proposition must be set out for all to see, and once that is done, our victim can do or not do what it says, as he sees fit.

It is a powerful argument, and one that logicians and

philosophers have apparently agreed to. It shows that even in a mechanistic universe, there is the situation that MacKay has called "a logical indeterminacy of a free choice." Although we tend to believe his point, our point is that while the formulation of the problem within the framework of a unitary consciousness may hold for each self, how does one apply it to multiple-self instances?

We are faced, it seems, with a new problem in analyzing the person. The person is a conglomeration of selves—a sociological entity. Because of our cultural bias toward language and its use, as well as the richness and flexibility that it adds to our existence, the governor of these multiple selves comes to be the verbal system. Indeed, a case can be made that the entire process of maturing in our culture is the process of the verbal system's trying to note and eventually control the behavioral impulses of the many selves that dwell inside of us.

Such a state of affairs makes the job for society and its judges extremely difficult. To which self do they mete out their punishments? As it stands, judges are, metaphorically speaking, called upon to punish the whole town for the wayward actions of one of its citizens. It is, of course, a poor solution, and in some sense, it may underlie the reason that punishment and rehabilitation rarely are effective in exercising behavioral control on a convicted felon. Just as social programs work poorly on a whole town because they are inherently unable to anticipate all the separate needs and conditions of its citizenry, the personal directive toward the person is equally sloppy and inaccurate in hitting the mark—the self that is responsible for the action in question.

REFERENCES

1. R. W. Sperry, 1969, A modified concept of consciousness, *Psychol. Rev.* 76:532–536.
2. J. C. Eccles, 1965, *The Brain and Unity of Conscious Experience, The 19th Arthur Stanley Eddington Memorial Lecture,* Cambridge, England: Cambridge University Press.

3. D. MacKay, 1972, Personal communication cited in M. S. Gazzaniga, One brain—Two minds? *Am. Sci. 60:*311–317.
4. J. E. LeDoux, D. H. Wilson, and M. S. Gazzaniga, 1977, A divided mind: Observations on the conscious properties of the separated hemispheres, *Annals of Neurology,* in press.
5. L. Festinger, 1957, *A Theory of Cognitive Dissonance,* Stanford, Calif. Stanford University Press.
6. G. L. Risse and M. S. Gazzaniga, 1976, Verbal retrieval of right hemisphere memories established in the absence of language, *Neurology 26:*354.
7. M. S. Gazzaniga, J. E. LeDoux, and D. H. Wilson, 1977, Language praxis and the right hemisphere: Clues to some mechanisms of consciousness, *Neurology,* in press.
8. S. Schachter, 1975, Cognition and peripheralist-centralist controversies in motivational emotion, in: M. S. Gazzaniga and C. Blakemore (Eds.), *Handbook of Psychobiology,* New York, Academic Press.
9. J. Klinger and P. Gloor, 1960, Connections of the amygdala and anterior commissure in the human brain, *J. Comp. Neurol. 115:*333–369.
10. M. S. Gazzaniga, 1966, Interhemispheric cuing systems remaining after section of neocortical commissures in monkeys, *Ext. Neurol. 16:*28–35.
11. M. S. Gazzaniga, 1966, Visuomotor integration in split-brain monkeys with other cerebral lesions, *Exp. Neurol. 16:*289–298.
12. M. S. Gazzaniga, 1970, *The Bisected Brain,* New York, Appleton-Century-Crofts.
13. C. Hamilton, 1974, Cross-cuing in monkeys, paper presented to Psychonometric Society, Boston.
14. C. Trevarthen, 1974, Functional relations of disconnected hemisphere with the brain stem and with each other: Monkey and man, in: W. L. Smith and M. Knosbourne (Eds.), *The Disconnected Cerebral Hemisphere and Behaviour,* Springfield, Ill., Charles C Thomas.
15. Garry Wills, 1964, *Politics and Catholic Freedom,* Chicago, Henry Regency Co.
16. D. MacKay, 1967, *Freedom of Action in a Mechanistic Universe, The Eddington Lecture,* Cambridge, England, Cambridge University Press.

Author Index

Acuna, C., 75
Akelaitis, A.J., 3, 21
Anker, R.L., 27, 43
Arrigoni, G., 73
Azulay, A., 43

Basser, L.S., 74, 99, 118
Battersby, N.S., 73
Beale, W., 99
Becker, W.A., 100
Bender, D.B., 40
Bender, M.B., 73
Bengston, L., 27, 42, 43
von Bergen, F.B., 100
Berlucchi, G., 40, 76, 118
Black, P., 42, 117
Blakemore, G., 40
Bogen, J.E., 3, 21, 43,
  46, 74, 83, 84, 88, 91,
  98, 100, 109, 114,
  115, 119
Bradshaw, J.L., 76
Brain, R., 72
Broca, P., 46
Brooks, L.R., 138
Brown, I.A., 100
Brown, J.W., 74, 75, 98
Branch, C., 99
Bremer, F., 42
Brinkman, S., 100
Burkland, C.W., 100, 118
Buschke, H., 110, 119
Butler, C.R., 40, 118

Carew, T.J., 41

Cartmill, M., 75
Choudhury, B.P., 39
Christopher, C., 44
Clark, E., 117
Collins, A., 138
Collins, R.L., 49
Collins, F., 75
Corballis, M., 99
Cragg, B.G., 27, 43
Crane, A.M., 138
Critchley, M., 72
Crosby, E.C., 41
Crow, T.J., 41
Culver, C., 7
Cuneod, M., 42

Darien-Smith, I., 43
Davenport, R.K., 119
DeAjuriaguerra, J., 72,
  75
Dennis, M., 75
DeRenzi, E., 73, 75, 76
Donchin, E., 67, 76
Doty, R.W., 40, 42
Durnford, M., 73

Eccles, J., 142, 161
Elberger, A., 27, 43
Ettlinger, G., 36, 44

Faglioni, P., 73, 75
Fellman, A., 100
Festinger, L., 162
Ford, R.F., 21, 42
Fox, C.A., 41

Francis, A., 27, 42, 43
Franco, L., 76
Freedman, H., 42, 117
French, L.A., 100
Fusella, A., 138

Galin, D., 67, 76
Gardner, A.K., 44
Gardner, W.J., 44
Gautier, J.C., 78, 98
Gazzaniga, M.S., 7, 40,
  41, 42, 43, 44, 46, 74,
  75, 76, 98, 99, 100,
  101, 117, 118, 119,
  126, 130, 138, 139,
  162
Geffen, G., 76
Georgopoulus, A., 75
Geschwind, N., 21, 42,
  91, 98, 100, 119, 139
Ghent, L., 73
Gibson, A., 41, 128,
  138
Gibson, J.J., 43, 56, 76
Glass, A., 74, 93, 94,
  95, 96, 101
Glickstien, M., 36, 44
Gloor, P., 42, 162
Gordon, P., 138
Green, D.M., 76
Gridlay, J.H., 44
Gross, C.G., 40
Gross, M.M., 76

Hallett, M., 42

Hamilton, C.R., 25, 40, 42, 43, 117, 118, 157, 158, 162
Heath, C.J., 43
Hebb, D.O., 123, 139
Hecaen, H., 72, 74, 75, 76, 98, 100
Henson, C.O., 37, 44
Hillyard, S., 99
Hirsch, H., 42
Hubel, D.H., 39, 43, 123
Hughes, R.A., 44
Hull, C., 138
Hume, P., 121, 138
Humphrey, T., 41
Hyvarinen, J., 75

Inhelder, B., 60, 75

Jackson, H., 46, 72
Jacobson, M., 42
James, M., 73
Jerison, H., 105, 118
Johnson, D., 100, 125, 138
Jones, E.G., 43, 119
Jones, F.W., 75
Jones, R.K., 79, 98
Jouandet, M., 100

Kahn, R.L., 73
Karnosh, L.J., 44
Karten, H., 42
Kerr, F.W.L., 43
Kimura, D., 65, 73, 76, 91, 100
Kinsbourne, M., 73
Kliest, K., 101
Kling, J.W., 40
Klinger, J., 42, 162
Kohn, B., 37, 44
Kuypers, H.G.J.M., 100

Lashley, K., 41, 103, 104, 117
Lauer, E.W., 41
LeCours, A., 99

LeDoux, J.E., 40, 41, 75, 76, 100, 111, 112, 113, 114, 117, 119, 138, 162
Lee-teng, E., 38, 44
LeGros Clark, W.E., 75
Leipmann, H., 91, 100
Levitsky, W., 98
Levine, M., 110
Levy, J., 44, 65, 66, 67, 74, 99
Lhermitte, F., 78, 98
Lomas, J., 100
Lynch, J.C., 75

MacCarty, C.S., 44
MacKay, D., 142, 160, 162
Maspes, P.E., 21, 42
Massonnet, J., 72
Matthew, W.D., 75
McBride, K.E., 46, 72
McClure, J.R., 44
McFie, J., 73
Meikle, T.H., 118
Menzel, E., 100
Milner, B., 52, 53, 73, 74, 99
Mishkin, M., 36, 40, 41, 43, 44, 118
Mitchell, D., 40
Morton, 36, 44
Mountcastle, V.B., 43, 44, 75
Myers, R., 1, 3, 11, 12, 26, 36, 37, 40, 41, 42, 43, 44, 117
Mukheries, S.K., 39

Nagylaki, T., 99
Nakamura, R., 101, 105, 106, 107, 108, 109, 118, 138
Nauta, W., 41, 42
Nebes, R., 53, 74
Negrao, N., 40
Neiderbuhl, J., 100

Neilsen, J.M., 72, 101
Neisser, U., 138
Nettleton, N.C., 76
Noble, J., 41
Nottebohm, F., 82, 83, 99

Ochs, S., 41
Olson, M., 99
Ornstein, R., 67, 76
Orton, S.T., 99
Overman, W.H., 42

Pandya, D.N., 42
Patterson, A., 72
Penfield, W., 83, 99
Petrinovich, L., 41
Piaget, J., 60, 75
Piercy, M., 73, 75
Pinsley, M., 148
Poggio, G.F., 43
Pollack, M., 73
Poranen, A., 75
Powell, T.P.S., 119
Preilowski, B.F.B., 44, 119
Premack, D., 74, 75, 92, 93, 94, 95, 96, 100, 101, 127, 128, 129, 138

Quillian, R., 138

Rakic, P., 100
Rasmussen, T., 99, 139
Reeves, A.G., 7
Riggs, L.A., 40
Risse, G.L., 14, 41, 43, 117, 119, 121, 131, 138, 162
Rizzolatti, G., 40
Roberts, L., 99
Robinson, J.S., 118
Rocha-Miranda, C.E., 40
Rogers, C.M., 119
Rose, J., 44
Rossing, H., 100
Russell, I.S., 41, 119

Sakata, H., 75
Schachter, S., 162
Schmitz, T., 41
Schneider, G.E., 62, 75
Schreiner, L.H., 44
Schwartz, A.S., 43
Schwartzman, R.J., 43
Scotti, G., 73
Sechzer, J.A., 118
Segal, S.J., 138
Semmes, J., 36, 43, 44, 73
Sheehan, P.W., 138
Skinner, B.F., 128, 129, 138
Smith, A., 74, 75, 99, 100, 118
Smith, G.E., 25
Smyth, J.O.G., 73
Sperry, R., 1, 3, 27, 36, 38, 41, 43, 44, 46, 65, 74, 76, 98, 99, 109, 110, 114, 141, 161

Spinnler, H., 73, 75, 76
Springer, S.P., 100, 117, 119
Stamm, J., 44
Sugar, O., 99, 118
Sullivan, M., 42, 117
Swets, J.A., 76
Szer, I.S., 138

Taylor, L., 52, 53, 74
Teuber, H.L., 73
Thompson, R., 41, 118
Treschner, J.H., 21, 42
Trevarthen, C., 65, 66, 67, 74, 158, 162

Vogel, P., 21, 46, 74, 100
Voneida, T.J., 118

Wada, J.A., 138
Wall, D.P., 43
Wallace, G., 76
Warrington, E.K., 73, 76

Washburn, S.L., 75
Weinstein, S., 73
Weschler, D., 119
Weisel, T., 39, 43, 123
Weisenberg, T., 46, 72
Wernicke, K., 46
White, R.H., 44
Whitlock, D.G., 42
Whitteridge, D., 39
Wilson, D.H., 6, 7, 21, 40, 75, 85, 100, 117, 119, 160, 162
Wilson, M.E., 39

Yakolev, 100
Yamaga, K., 40

Zaidel, D., 44, 109, 110, 114, 119
Zaidel, E., 74, 84, 99
Zangwill, O., 72, 73, 75, 99
Zeki, S.M., 42

Subject Index

alexia without agraphia, 23
amygdala, 153
amytal, 14, 81, 131, 150
angiography, 14, 131, 150
aphasia, 93, 96, 97
  global, 96, 97
attitudes, 155
attribution, 146-151, 154
auditory transfer, 23

bimanual motor coordination, *see* motor coordination
binocular depth perception, *see* depth perception
block design, 48, 67

callosotomy, 114, 116, 117, 122, 123
chimeric stimuli, 65-67
cognitive capacity, 103-117
cognitive dissonance, 150, 155-157
commissural sensory window, 11, 13, 117
commissural system, *see* commissures, forebrain
commissural transmission limits, 11, 12
commissure, anterior, 3, 6, 9, 10, 20-23, 25, 26, 122, 153, 154
commissures
  forebrain, 2, 9, 10, 11, 13, 16, 17, 19, 24, 25, 108, 116, 123, 125
  tectal, 24
commissurotomy, cerebral (forebrain), 6, 17, 21, 39, 103, 104, 109, 110, 115
consciousness, 5, 124, 131, 134, 141-161
  animal, 145

corpus callosum, 1, 2, 3, 6, 9, 10, 11, 12, 21, 22, 23, 131, 153
  body, 2
  genus, 2
  rostrum, 2
  splenium, 2, 12, 21, 23, 25, 26, 28, 29
cross-cuing, 38, 157
cube drawing, 51, 52
cuing, 34-39, *see also* cross-cuing

decussation, 10, 24, 25
depth perception, 18
digit span task, 110
dorsal column, 30-39

emotion, 151-155
  cognitive theory, 151-155
emotional encoding, 151-155
engram, 11, 13, 14, 15, 91
  transfer, 13-17, 125, *see also* transfer of training, interhemispheric
epilepsy, 3, 109, 115, 122
equipotentiality, 103, 104

face agnosia, 71
fragmented figures, 53, 54, 64
free will, 159-161

handedness, 92
hemispherectomy, 36, 88, 90, 106, 108
homolateral somatosensory representation, 29, 36, 37, 58, 91
homologous brain areas, 24, 25, 104
homotopic connections, 16, 116
hypothesis task, 110-115

imagery, 121-124
intelligence, 103-117
interhemispheric communication, 9-44,
    104, 117, 125
interhemispheric transfer, *see* interhemis-
    pheric communication
intermanual transfer, 29-39
interocular transfer, 2
ipsilateral cuing, 37, *see also* homo-
    lateral somatosensory representation

language, 58-63, 73, 77-101
    artificial, 92-96
    and consciousness, 141-161
    development, 78-83, 92
    lateralization, 78-83
    natural, 92-96
    metal, 93-96
    right hemisphere, 83
lateralization, 45-76
learning, errorless, 125-129
limbic system, 17, 20, 153, 154

manipulospatiality, 18, 55-76
mass action, 103-108
medial leniniscus, 30-39
memory, 124-137
    associative, 136, 137
    encoding of, 130-137
    multidimensionality of, 130-137
    short term, 106-110
    systems, 135-137
    theory, 135-137
metalanguage, 93-96
mood, 154
motivation, 125-129
motor coordination, 18, 117
motor transfer, 16

neglect, 69

olfactory transfer, 23, 153
optic chiasm, 1, 2, 11, 105

pain, *see* somatosensation
personal responsibility, 159-161
praxis, 91-92
proprioception, *see* somatosensation
prosopagnosia, 71
psycholinguistics, 96

recall, 136
recognition, 136
reinforcement, 125-129
rewards, 125-129

selective reminding in free recall task,
    110
self-image, 155
sensorimotor efficiency, 117
sensorimotor functions, 104, 108, 150
sensorimotor losses, 104-108
sensory—sensory integration, 116, 117
sodium amytal, *see* amytal
somatosensation, 29-39
specialization, 45-76
spinothalamic tract, 30-39
spreading depression, cortical, 13-14
stereognosis, *see* somatosensation
syntax, 84

temperature, *see* somatosensation
touch, *see* somatosensation
transfer of training, interhemispheric,
    13, *see also* interhemispheric com-
    munication

unilateral spatial agnosia, 69

values, 155
visual imagery, *see* imagery
visual transfer, 19-23

Wechsler Adult Intelligence Scale
    (W.A.I.S.), 110
Wechsler Memory Scale, 110, 111
wire figures, 52